Current
Feminist Issues
in
Psychotherapy

Current Feminist Issues in Psychotherapy

Guest Editors
The New England Association for Women in Psychology

Women & Therapy
Volume 1, Number 3

The Haworth Press
New York

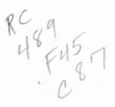

The Haworth Press, Inc., 28 East 22 Street, New York, NY 10010.

Library of Congress Cataloging in Publication Data
Main entry under title:

Current feminist issues in psychotherapy.

(Women & therapy ; v. 1, no. 3)
Includes bibliographical references.
1. Feminist therapy—Addresses, essays, lectures. 2. Women—Mental health—Addresses, essays, lectures. I. New England Association for Women in Psychology. II. Series. [DNLM: 1. Psychotherapy. 2. Women's rights. 3. Women. W1 WO433V v.1 no.3 / WM 420 C975]
RC489.F45C87   1982   616.89'14'088042   82-15721
ISBN 0-86656-206-0

Current Feminist Issues in Psychotherapy

Women & Therapy
Volume 1, Number 3

CONTENTS

Current
Feminist Issues
in
Psychotherapy

EDITORIAL

I am excited to introduce the first special issue of *Women & Therapy,* *"Current Feminist Issues in Psychotherapy."* A working committee of members of the New England Association for Women in Psychology has organized this issue. The selected articles deal with topics of deep significance to women.

The first issue of *Women & Therapy* arrived from the printer this week. It is impressive with several articles written by members of the journal's editorial board. *Women & Therapy* is, indeed, a collective effort with active participation by the editorial board in writing, soliciting articles, and reviewing manuscripts. We are eager to receive more manuscripts from women who have made life changes through their experiences in therapy!

This is the last issue to be published in 1982, a year of increasing political activity. As I write this, anti-nuclear demonstrations are being held in major cities throughout the world. As Britain and Argentina fight in the Falkland Islands, many of us are organizing against war, against bombs, against military solutions to human problems. As feminists who believe in the power of people to change, it is time to speak out against destructive forces and demonstrate to the world how to resolve conflict in non-violent ways.

Betts Collett

May 1982

1

INTRODUCTION

The Association for Women in Psychology (AWP) began as a formal organization in 1969 in order to address the following goals:

a. Ending the role psychology has had in perpetuating unscientific and unquestioned assumptions about the "natures" of women and men;
b. Encouraging feminist psychological research on sex and gender;
c. Encouraging research and theory directed towards alternatives to stereotyped sex roles, child-raising practices, non-sexist life-styles and new vocabularies.

The 1981 National Conference of AWP had the theme "Feminism in the 80s: Weaving New Connections." Indeed, as a result of the enthusiasm engendered by these new connections, a New England chapter of AWP was formed in the summer of 1981. The Publications Committee, which constitutes the guest editors of this special issue, first met to discuss publishing some of the material presented at the conference. A call for abstracts elicited a wide variety of topics on issues in feminist therapy, and this variety is reflected by the articles in this issue.

The contents of this issue include clinical issues, such as depression, battered women, sibling incest, and women with physical and developmental disabilities; and issues that address women's socialization, such as single-parent women-headed households, the black sisterhood, displaced homemakers, women's body image, and women's career decision-making processes. The authors include therapists, consultants, educators, researchers, and students, thus representing the range of interests of women in psychology. The special issue has contributions by women who have published widely in their fields as well as by new writers. Some of the topics in this special issue have rarely before been addressed in a professional journal. We realize that this issue omits many other important topics, such as the problems in living facing older women, Lesbians, and Hispanic women, to mention just a few examples. Hopefully, this will be the agenda of further issues of this journal.

This issue goes to the publisher the same month as the first New England AWP Conference on the Psychology of Women takes place, with the theme "Women Helping Women: Research, Therapy and Politics." For the editors, this publishing project has spanned the time between the two conferences and provided a means of promoting research and thinking on feminist therapy. For the reader of this issue, we hope to stimulate further collection of data and ideas as they affect women's lives.

Guest Editors (in alphabetical order)
    Fraelean Curtis
    Margaret Downes
    Marcia Germaine Hutchinson
    Dorothy McIntosh
    Jill V. Richard
    Esther D. Rothblum
    Gail Washor-Liebhaber

WOMEN'S SOCIALIZATION AND THE PREVALENCE OF DEPRESSION: THE FEMININE MISTAKE

Esther D. Rothblum

Depression is one of the most prevalent psychiatric disorders existing today. Although most people feel down, "blue," or depressed as the result of common stresses of living, a "clinical" depression is more severe than a temporary sad mood. The *Diagnostic and Statistical Manual* of the American Psychiatric Association (DSM-III, 1980) defines a major depressive episode to consist of three criteria:

1. a dysphoric mood or loss of interest and pleasure is present and relatively persistent;
2. at least four of the eight symptoms of poor appetite or weight loss, insomnia or increased sleep, psychomotor agitation or retardation, loss of interest in usual activities, loss of energy or fatigue, feelings of worthlessness, diminished concentration, and suicidal ideation, are present every day for at least two weeks; and
3. there is no evidence of mania, psychosis, organic mental disorder or normal bereavement.

In particular, women consistently present higher rates of depression than men, usually at a ratio of two-to-one. Not only are women more likely than men to enter treatment following depression, but studies that randomly survey communities find more depressed women than depressed men in the general population (Weissman & Klerman, 1977). The life-time risk for developing depression ranges from 2 percent to 12 percent for men and from 5 percent to 26 percent for women (Boyd & Weissman, in press). Suicide rates, however, are higher for men than for women, although more women than men attempt suicide.

Esther D. Rothblum is a clinical psychologist in New Haven, CT. She is co-editor of the book *The Stereotyping of Women: Its Effects on Mental Health*.

I. Biological Versus Environmental Factors

The sex difference in depression rates has lead researchers to postulate greater biological susceptibility among women for depression. In the most complete review to date, Weissman and Klerman (1977) have investigated the evidence for possible genetic transmission and for female endocrine physiological processes. The evidence they cite concerning the relationship between depression and endocrinological factors is inconsistent. There is very good evidence that depression increases during the postpartum period. The evidence for premenstrual tension and for depression as the result of oral contraceptives is inconsistent. Finally, there is very good evidence that menopause does not result in higher depression rates. Thus, there is insufficient evidence that the two-to-one ratio of women to men in depression rates is accounted for by biological factors.

Several environmental factors have been postulated to account for the high rates of depression among women. First, women's roles may be more restricted than men's and allow for less financial, social, or occupational gratification. Secondly, women may be socialized to be unassertive, dependent, and passive, all of which lead to depression rather than action under stress. Thirdly, as the media increasingly present exceptional women who have "made it" in high-level careers, many women may feel depressed with their own inability to meet these rising expectations. Finally, women may be taught to be helpless and to experience a lack of control over their environment, so that the perception of no relationship between their efforts and any significant results would lead to depression.

II. Research on Women and Depression

The research on societal factors and on women's roles that could relate to depression will be reviewed. Specifically, this review will focus on the societal roles of social networks, marriage, divorce and separation, housework versus full-time employment, and parenthood. Emphasis will be on the differential effects of these roles on women and men. For a more complete review, see Rothblum (1982).

Lack of social networks and supports, especially the lack of a meaningful intimate relationship, is a major risk factor for depression among both women and men. However, there is some evidence that women are more affected than men by the absence of such social supports. Depression in men is more often associated with competency-related issues (such as loss of a job); depression in women is more often related to less warmth and expressiveness (such as the break-up of a relationship; Chevron, Quinlan, & Blatt, 1978). Women are also more likely than men to experience depression following rejection or distance in a relationship (Parker, 1980).

Marriage affects women and men in different ways. Married men are less depressed than never-married men whereas married women are more depressed than those who never married (Gove, 1972; Radloff, 1975; Radloff & Rae, 1979). Furthermore, depressed married women have more marital problems than non-depressed women (Bullock, Siegel, Weissman, & Paykel, 1972).

One speculation regarding depression rates and marital status is that married women are more likely than never-married women to be homemakers and thus to occupy a position that has come to be regarded as boring, unrewarding and unprestigious (Gove, 1972). Lack of paid employment does predispose women to depression (Brown & Harris, 1978). Furthermore, depressed women who were not employed tended to experience more marital friction and to be less satisfied with their work than employed married women (Weissman, Paykel, Siegel, & Klerman, 1971).

Another speculation concerning high depression rates for married women is that employed wives carry the major burden of child care and housework in addition to their jobs. In order to investigate this theory, Radloff (1975) analyzed amount of housework that married men and women engaged in. Her results indicate that 23 percent of husbands "work around the house or yard every day" compared with 69 percent of employed wives and 80 percent of housewives. Thus, employed wives engage in nearly as much housework as housewives do, indicating a dual load of work.

Marital disruption is more likely to occur for women than for men since women are less likely to remarry following divorce and since women are more likely to be widows as a result of living longer than men and marrying men who are older than themselves. Among all categories of marital status, depression rates are highest for separated and divorced women (Hirschfeld & Cross, 1980).

An analysis of the course of depression among divorced women and men (Briscoe & Smith, 1973) indicated that women were more depressed during the marriage whereas men became depressed at the time of the marital separation. More women than men had depressive symptoms that were related to specific precipitating events, such as being informed of the spouse's adultery or the spouse's request for a divorce. Briscoe and Smith's study thus indicates that depressed divorced men and women constitute different samples. Women are more likely to become depressed in a disrupted marriage, often as the result of specific events contributing to the marital friction. Few demographic variables distinguish depressed women from their nondepressed counterparts, suggesting that it is the events leading to divorce that also result in depression. Divorced men, on the other hand, have a history of precipitating interpersonal and sexual factors that is not present among non-depressed divorced men. This suggests that among men, the incapacitating symptoms of depression may result in divorce.

Parenthood is a time of major responsibilities and stress. Parents with young children at home constitute a high percentage of depressed individuals (Shapiro, Parry, & Brewin, 1979; Brown & Harris, 1978).

Not only do women assume the majority of child care responsibilities, as mentioned previously, but over 85 percent of single parents are women (Brandwein, Brown & Fox, 1974). Single mothers are faced with difficulties that range from financial problems and problems with childrearing to loneliness and the stress of socialization. Ilgenfritz (1961) identified fear of loneliness, loss of self-esteem, practical problems of living and specific concerns for children as the major stresses facing single mothers attending a parent education program.

Contrary to popular belief, women do not tend to experience "the empty nest syndrome." Rather than becoming depressed when grown children leave the home, women in this age group are low on depression (Radloff, 1980).

Full-time employment is related to satisfaction among women (Hall & Gordon, 1972) and employed women who were depressed recover faster in treatment than homemakers (Mostow & Newberry, 1975).

There has been little research on women in *nontraditional roles*, such as professional or executive women. Welner et al., (Welner, Martin, Wochnick, Davis, Fishman & Clayton, 1979) investigated psychiatric illness among women physicians and PhDs in the community. Their results indicated that 51 percent of women physicians and 32 percent of women PhDs had primary affective disorders. Their study found little evidence of other forms of psychiatric illnesses. Sixty-seven percent of depressed women physicians and 70 percent of depressed women PhDs reported prejudice in their training or employment; the figures for non-depressed physicians and PhDs were 50 percent and 48 percent, respectively. Thus, prejudice was reported significantly more often by the depressed women. Similarly, Pitts, Schuller, Rich and Pitts (1979) examined the American Medical Association records of deaths of physicians. They found the suicide rate for women physicians to be 6.56 percent, higher than that of male physicians and four times higher than the suicide rate for white American females of the same age. Although additional research is needed to corroborate these findings, it appears that professional women are a significantly higher risk for depression and suicide.

In society, it is more acceptable for women than men to *express depression*. Hammen and Peters (1978) used both male and female college students to rate male and female confederates who played a standardized, depressed or nondepressed role over the telephone. Results showed that depressed persons of the opposite sex were most strongly rejected. Female raters made little distinction between depressed males and females on role impairment. Male raters, however, considered the depressed females more impaired.

Finally, there is some evidence that men make better use of *coping skills* in/the face of stressful life events than women do (Pearlin & Schooler, 1978). Thus, women are not only at higher risk for depression but they seem to receive less preparation to cope with disruptive life events.

Rothblum (1982) concludes that "Basically, the woman who hopes for marriage, a family, and a providing husband who will be the sole wage-earner, is dramatically increasing her chances of depression. On the other hand, the woman who enters graduate or medical school to pursue an advanced degree traditionally reserved for men is not immune from stress and depression" as a result of the prejudice and sexism in these professions. Thus rates of depression and suicide among professional women are extremely high. It is evident that depression among women in significantly affected by women's sex roles regarding work, the marital relationship, and motherhood. In general, societal roles place women at greater risk for depression than men.

III. Therapy for Depressed Women

Traditional forms of treatment for depression include pharmacotherapy, in the form of antidepressant medication, and psychotherapy, such as psychodynamic psychotherapy, behavior therapy, family therapy, and marital therapy. There is little doubt that these therapies are effective for alleviating depression among both women and men (see Weissman, 1981 for a review of therapy efficacy). Much has been written criticizing traditional forms of therapy for women (see Al-Issa, 1980; Howell & Bayes, 1981; Brodsky & Hare-Mustin, 1980; Rawlings & Carter, 1977). Critics of pharmacotherapy state that drugs alleviate the symptoms but not the cause of depression among women and "tend to explain female life problems in psychiatric terms" (Al-Issa, 1980, p. 42). Feminists have criticized psychoanalytic theory as being phallocentric and humiliating to women (Howell & Bayes, 1981), and psychotherapy as aimed "to help the woman patient achieve this resignation—to accept her femininity as compensatory, as second best" (Menaker, 1974, p.232). Behavior therapy, it has been pointed out, may focus on reinforcing the depressed female patient for engaging in the very domestic or sex-role stereotyped tasks that triggered the depression (Al-Issa, 1980).

There has been much confusion surrounding the term *feminist therapy*. The Federations of Professional Women (1981) have described feminist therapy to include (p.27):

1. A more egalitarian relationship between the client and therapist.
2. An understanding of the effects of sexism, discrimination, and sex role socialization on the development and maintenance of problems in women and men.
3. Encouragement of expanded role options for women and men.

These criteria may not readily distinguish feminist therapists from experienced therapists in general. However, feminist therapy incorporates strategies of social change for women in addition to individual change. Thus, change at the community or organizational level may be the most effective source of education, intervention, and prevention. Several strategies will be presented for decreasing depression among women that incorporate both feminist therapy as a means of treatment and of changing societal roles as a means of prevention for depression.

The preceding section has identified the relationship of significant others with depression among women. It would seem evident that *marital therapy*, *family therapy*, or other means of involving partners in the process of therapy is an effective intervention. Specifically, therapy should focus on domestic, child care, and occupational roles of both spouses or partners. Rather than maintain the traditional structure of the family, therapist and clients should examine more flexible and nontraditional alternatives. Hare-Mustin (1981) suggests redefining the responsibilities of family members, equalizing power, questioning sex role stereotypes in relationships, and negotiating a "contract" that states the goals of therapy.

Group therapy would seem indicated for depressed women given the frequency of the diagnosis. In addition to cost-effectiveness, a group setting allows individual women to share experiences and to recognize commonalities, as well as to receive support and encouragement from the group members. Finally, the group serves a social function by decreasing the social isolation and lack of activity often experienced by depressed individuals.

Specific *skills training* may be appropriate for depressed women given the varied and complex antecedents to depression. Assertion training has been recommended for depressed women given women's socialization to be passive and helpless under stress. Social skills training can be effective to increase social support networks and to increase the quality of interpersonal relationships. Career counseling is helpful for women with limited employment histories or lack of information about organizational factors. Time management counseling may aid women who have difficulty delegating responsibility, prioritizing work, and otherwise feel overwhelmed by daily schedules.

Unfortunately, clients who enter therapy for depression are not in an ideal situation to embark on major life changes. They are, by virtue of their depressed mood, at their most passive and fatigued, with little energy or activity level. Secondly, self-confidence and optimism that changes will succeed are low. Finally, it is difficult to provide strategies of intervention for clients *after* the divorce or the termination of a job rather than while clients are still in a position to effect change. Thus, community prevention measures are a highly preferable strategy for depression.

Educational programs should be developed for schools, community organizations and business settings to increase awareness of risk factors for depression, sex role stereotypes about women's roles, and demographic and societal changes that affect women. The media in particular have changed the public's awareness of depression as the topic appears in newspapers and magazines, and is discussed on television and radio talk shows.

Changing, consulting with, and advising institutions concerning existing practices that increase depression for women is a means of primary prevention. Setting up programs in work settings that bring together individuals with similar difficulties, such as working mothers with young children or women in nontraditional careers, is an effective way of providing awareness of support. Increasing numbers of women are entering the work force or returning to school to complete degrees. These women and their employers are pointing out the problems encountered as institutions traditionally comprised mainly of men struggle to incorporate women.

Training health professionals regarding the extensiveness of depression among women, societal risk factors that precede depression among women, are effective intervention strategies. Training professionals is a cost-effective manner of effective large-scale change.

Given the high prevalence rates of depression among women, treatment and prevention programs for depressed women and for women at risk for depression should constitute a high priority. In light of current data on women's roles and on mental health practices, failure to prioritize research and treatment on depressed women will not only maintain the high prevalence rates in the coming decade, but increase them.

REFERENCES

Al-Issa, I. *The Psychopathology of Women*. Englewood Cliffs, NJ: Prentice-Hall, 1980.

Boyd, J. H. & Weissman, M. M. The epidemiology of affective disorders. *Archives of General Psychiatry*, in press.

Brandwein, R. A., Brown, C. A., & Fox, E. M. Women and children last: The social situation of divorced mothers and their families. *Journal of Marriage and the Family*, 1974, *36*, 498–514.

Briscoe, C. W., & Smith, J. B. Depression and marital turmoil. *Archives of General Psychiatry*, 1973, *29*, 811–817.

Brodsky, A. M., & Hare-Mustin, R. (Eds.) *Women and Psychotherapy*. New York: Guilford Press, 1980.

Brown, G. W., & Harris, T. O. *Social Origins of Depression*. London, England: Tavistock, 1978.

Bullock, R. C., Siegel, R., Weissman, M. M., & Paykel, E. S. The weeping wife: Marital relations of depressed women. *Journal of Marriage and the Family*, 1972, August, 488–495.

Chevron, E. S., Quinlan, D. M., & Blatt, S. J. Sex roles and gender differences in the experiences of depression. *Journal of Abnormal Psychology*, 1978, *87*, 680–683.

Federations of Professional Women. *Women and Psychotherapy: A Consumer Handbook*. 1981.

Gove, W. R. The relationship between sex roles, marital status and mental illness. *Social Forces*, 1972, *51*, 34–44.

Hall, D. T., & Gordon, F. E. Career choices of married women: Effects on conflict role behavior and satisfaction. *Journal of Applied Psychology*, 1973, *58*, 42–48.

Hammen, D. L., & Peters, S. D. Interpersonal consequences of depression: Responses to men and women enacting a depressed role. *Journal of Abnormal Psychology*, 1978, *87*, 322–332.

Hirschfeld, R. M. A., & Cross, C. H. Psychosocial risk factors for depression. In: Regier, D. A., & Allen, G. (Eds.) *Risk Factor Research in the Major Mental Disorders*. National Institutes of Mental Health. DHHS Pub. No. (ADM) 81-1068, Washington, D. C.: Supt. of Docs., U.S. Govt. Print. Off., 1981.

Howell, E., & Bayes, M. (Eds.) *Women and Mental Health*. New York: Basic Books, 1981.

Ilgenfritz, M. P. Mothers on their own: Widows and divorcees. *Marriage and Family Living*. 1961, *23*, 38–41.

Menaker, E. In Franks, V., & Burtle, V. (Eds.) *Women in Therapy*. New York: Brunner/Mazel, 1974.

Mostow, E., & Newberry, P. Work role and depression in women: A comparison of workers and housewives in treatment. *American Journal of Orthopsychiatry*, 1975, *45*, 538–548.

Pearlin, L. J., & Schooler, C. The structure of coping. *Journal of Health and Social Behavior*, 1978, *19*, 2–21.

Pitts, F. N., Schuller, B., Rich, C. L., & Pitts, A. F. Suicide among U.S. women physicians, 1967–1972. *American Journal of Psychiatry*, 1979, *136*, 694–696.

Radloff, L. Sex differences in depression: The effects of occupation and marital status. *Sex Roles*, 1975, *1*, 249–265.

Radloff, L. Depression and the empty nest. *Sex Roles*, 1980, *6*, 775–781.

Radloff, L., & Rae, D. S. Susceptibility and precipitating factors in depression: Sex differences and similarities. *Journal of Abnormal Psychology*, 1979, *88*, 174–181.

Rawlings, E. I., & Carter, D. K. (Eds.) *Psychotherapy for Women: Treatment Toward Equality*. Springfield, Il: Charles C Thomas, 1977.

Rothblum, E. D. Sex role stereotypes and depression in women. In Franks, V., & Rothblum, E. D. (Eds.) *The Stereotyping of Women: Its Effects on Mental Health*. New York: Springer Publishing Co., in press.

Shapiro, D. A., Parry, G., & Brewin, C. Stress, coping and psychotherapy: The foundations of a clinical approach. In Cox, T., & Mackay, C. (Eds.) *Psychophysiological Response to Occupational Stress*. International Publishing Co., 1979.

Weissman, M. M. Antidepressants and psychotherapy in depression. *Advances in Biological Psychiatry*, 1981, *7*, 230–239.

Weissman, M. M., & Klerman, G. L. Sex differences and the epidemiology of depression. *Archives of General Psychiatry*, 1977, *34*, 98–111.

Weissman, M. M., Paykel, E. S., Siegel, R., & Klerman, G. L. The social role performance of depressed women: Comparisons with a normal group. *American Journal of Orthopsychiatry*, 1971, *41*, 390–405.

Welner, A., Martin, S., Wochnick, E., Davis, M. A., Fishman, R., & Clayton, P. J. Psychiatric disorders among professional women. *Archives of General Psychiatry*, 1979, *36*, 169–172.

ADDRESSING STRESS FACTORS IN SINGLE-PARENT WOMEN-HEADED HOUSEHOLDS

Jill V. Richard

Introduction

Formerly referrred to as divorced, widowed or unwed mothers, women who raise children without husbands are most currently being referred to as what they are, ''Single-Parent Mothers,'' rather than what they are no longer. Beyond circumventing the judgements that are implied by defining a woman in terms of her lost status, ''single-parent'' defines the identity of a group that can be observed and compared to other groups. This unified and affirmative group status allows an observer to compare these parents to others and question the basis for inequities in economic and social status, as well as in other areas. Current statistics on single-parent women, suggest that overall, single-parent families, headed by women endure economic hardships unmatched by two-parent families and perhaps also by their male counterparts.

This author's clinical experience also suggests that the economic, social and emotional problems encountered by female single-parents differ from those of male-single parents. A therapeutic model will be presented which addresses the needs of single-parent, women clients. Strategies which attack the root of the problem are also discussed.

Statistics

The stress factors that single-parent mothers deal with daily may be invisible to the clinician, and she/he may assume that the mother is inordinately depressed, anxious and passive. The client may appear unmotivated, inef-

Ms. Richard is a Psychiatric Social Worker for a public school system, south of Boston. She provides family, individual and couples therapy, as well as parent education to the families of pre-school and school-aged children.

15

fective and uncaring about her children. The following statistics begin to shed some light on the plight of single-parent, women-headed families.

According to the Bureau of the Census, in 1978, 14 percent of 57.2 million families were maintained by a woman with no husband present. From another perspective, "about 10 million or 17 percent of children were living in families which did not include a father, as compared with only 1.5 percent in families which were maintained without a mother." (Bureau of the Census, August 1978).

How did these female-headed households support themselves financially? Though more than 50 percent of these women participated in the labor force in 1976, approximately 75 percent received part of their income in the form of transfer payments (i.e., public assistance and Supplemental Security Income). Men who were receiving financial assistance through transfer payments had a median income of $9,430, while women in the same category had a median income of $3,580. (Bureau of the Census, April 1978).

Despite dual sources of income for 25–50 percent of female-headed families, the median income in 1976 was $7,210 as compared to $16,200 for husband-wife families. In 1976, the median income for all families was $14,960. For white families, the median income was $15,540, as compared to Blacks at $9,240 and Spanish at $10,260. (Bureau of the Census, April 1978). These figures suggest that it is probable that female minority heads of families are likely to be suffering further hardships.

In 1976, the total poverty population consisted of 25 million people. Husband-wife families accounted for 6 percent of that total. Female-headed families represented 36 percent of the poverty population, though they only accounted for 11 percent of the general population. This means that female-headed households were three times over represented in the poverty sector, more than any other identified poverty population (Black, Spanish and the aged). (Bureau of the Census, April 1978). This clearly demonstrates that poverty is more rampant among female-headed families than among other commonly acknowledged poverty-prone populations.

A recent *"Newsweek"* Magazine article reports that nearly half of poor families are headed by women. "This feminization of poverty...accounts for virtually all the growth in the poverty rolls since 1970—a scarifying 53 percent increase that shows no sign of slowing as out-of-wedlock birth and divorce rates continue to soar." According to the President's National Advisory Council on Economic Opportunity, "If the trend continues,...the poverty population would be composed solely of women and their children before the year 2000." (*"Newsweek,"* April 5, 1982).

What we are looking at, then, is a massive, unidentified social problem which needs to be addressed at the federal and state levels. Other identified poverty populations have helped by specifically targeted government programs designed to improve their standard of living. The largest decline in the number of low-income elders took place in 1969–76 when substantial increases in social security benefits were enacted. The portion of the poverty population represented by the aged declined from 20 percent in 1969 to 13 percent in 1976. This statement suggests that government policies can have major impact on the standard of living for certain identified poverty groups. It is evident that current family legislation is non-supportive of a viable single-parent lifestyle for women and their children.

Clinical Issues

The reader might wonder why one would attempt to deal with what is essentially a social problem as a clinical issue, or how one would approach this. Delinquency and child abuse are social issues that also require large scale solutions. Yet, because they are complex problems and because their solution is not the highest governmental priority, much of the work must be done at the individual level. To restore many individuals to healthy functioning is more difficult than to address the factors that interfere with healthy emotional growth and adjustment. As clinicians we do not have the option of preventing the problem. We can, however, offer assistance to people attempting to cope with their circumstances.

Since we cannot individually eradicate the social forces causing the stresses single-parent mothers face, we deal clinically with their economic and psychological impact on the individual. In the economic realm alone, financial problems for these women translate into clinical issues in that economic problems: 1. Demand better than average coping skills, 2. Lead to problems that become social in nature, such as housing, health care and child care, 3. These, in turn, lead to problems that become emotional in nature; for example, lowered self-esteem, anxiety and guilt.

These three types of problems and the economic basis for them need to be sorted out in order for the clinician and the client to begin to address them. Though lack of money is a factor which induces and increases stress for women-headed families, other issues, such as difficulty in coping with social stigma or anxiety and guilt regarding parenting, may appear as clinical issues and be unrelated to the client's financial status.

Differences Between Single-Parent Mothers' and Fathers' Living Circumstances

Of great interest to this author was the clinical phenomenon that single-parent fathers lived in very different circumstances than single-parent mothers. The single-parent fathers in this author's small clinical sample had adequate income for their needs. They continued to work a full eight hour day or longer. They had women, either relatives or paid neighbors, who provided affordable or no cost child care which allowed fathers to maintain a fairly well-paying job. Thus, their income allowed them to maintain their previous role and to replace their wife's role with the children for the time they were at work. In addition, they were able to live in the same residence and maintain a standard of living that was relatively similar to the one that they had had as a dual parent family. Fathers did not experience the trauma of entering the job market, or lack of adequate work, nor were they required to adjust to the role of full-time child care provider.

The major adjustments for fathers on entering their single-parent role were probably emotional. It appeared that most single-parent fathers tended to continue to maintain a similar lifestyle to the situation pre-loss or divorce of the wife, except that they had to make adjustments to the divorce or loss and make adjustments in their social life. (In comparison, single-parent women tended to withdraw from social contact.) Two other areas that demanded the father's attention were: 1. The children's unconscious expectations and demands for the father to take on more of the nurturing role, 2. The community holding the father more accountable for the welfare of the child and the overall daily care of the child and, to a lesser degree, the home. It also seemed that relatives or perhaps adequate income allowed for some of the house chores to be done by others.

Fathers generally appeared so unfamiliar with the nurturing role, particularly the emotionally related aspects, that they tended to overlook many aspects of the job unless prodded by the community or the children themselves. Yet, emotional nurturance is an area of child care, which if overlooked, may not be immediately evident to an outside observer. Conflict arose in situations where the child's needs, such as illness, interfered with the father's job or his perception of his role at home. Generally though, fathers appeared to either have a child care situation that was flexible enough to cover for him or he would allow the child to stay home alone. Conflict might come from outside the family when the neighbors or school felt the latter was an inadequate solution. Evenings and weekends for these fathers with school-age children probably required more of their focus and involvement. It appeared, though, that the father's conception of the child's nurturant needs would probably have been less than a mother's in the same position. It would be difficult to assess the impact of the change from dual to single-parent status, since for the male most of the major adjustments appear to occur on the emotional level.

The clinical sample of single-parent fathers is too small to fully illuminate the issues involved. Beyond the need for some specific parenting skills, it appears that most of the adjustments are confined to the specific changes in the single-parent male's roles of spouse and father. They appear not to severely impair his self concept, nor to invade other aspects of his life.

For female single-parents (and the majority of those single parents I saw were mothers) the issues were different. In every case but perhaps one, money was an issue at the survival level. Beyond survival, lack of access to money left women in circular traps with no options and no relief. Though these women appeared to emotionally react to feeling trapped, they often appeared too overwhelmed to consciously recognize the full-cycle of the traps without the assistance of an outsider.

One of the most basic needs of single-parent mothers is for a job that provides a viable income. Yet, if no public transportation is available, as is the case with these women, they need a car to get a decent paying job. Conversely, they need a decent paying job in order to afford transportation to that job. They also need child care in order to get a job to pay for the child care. They may even need money to get training or education in order to obtain a job that will lift the family out of poverty. In addition, because they are single parents, they require more flexible jobs than seem to be available to them. They often require local, perhaps part-time work, that allows them to care for a sick child or to contact their children during the day. Most jobs do not allow for this, particularly the unskilled or semi-skilled ones which appear to be the type generally offered to them.

While trapped in one area, women can find no relief in other areas. Beyond its survival function, money also buys relief in many other realms. Money buys relief from anxiety about finances and from the tentativeness of a living situation, safer neighborhoods, better schools, the whims of ever-changing welfare roles and regulations, recreation for a child, easier transportation and generally fewer everyday problems. Money also buys options. For families existing at or just above the poverty level, few dollars are available to meet their family's basic needs. When crises or chronic problems develop, these families have few or no choices. They are unable to mobilize their resources to meet the crisis, without threatening their survival in other critical areas, such as rent, food, heat, and electricity. Money offers the adult a sense of choice and control, a sense of being less passive in meeting her own and her family's needs. For these women, lack of money meant lack of control of their own lives.

Lack of money also caused other forms of inner conflict. Women experienced guilt and anxiety when they could not provide for their children. Due to socialization in this culture, mothers are expected (and expect themselves) to nurture their children, regardless of their emotional or material ability to do so. Though single-parent males received support from neighbors and relatives, single-parent women seemed to be expected to provide materially and nurture consistently without help. Unlike men, single-parent women seemed to be solely responsible for 24 hours a day child care. When they were unable to "handle it" they questioned their own parenting ability. Guilt and anxiety over parenting only added to their stress. The increased stress taxed their ability to parent well.

These women on welfare or in low paying jobs seemed to have few family supports, few family members in a position to offer help and few professional contacts that could assist them without a fee. Overwhelmed by problems, they appeared to have little energy and few resources to barter.

With no money and no relief from parenting there was no way for these women to buy "time off" in order to reduce stress or gain a new perspective. They were only further demoralized by their unacknowledged plight and the lack of options available to them. Socialization resulting in passivity and dependence in the face of stress only complicated their difficulties. Further barriers resulted from discriminatory attitudes and practices that are aimed at women in general, and at female-single parents.

How might the single-parent mother appear to a clinician in the office? Perhaps she would appear overwhelmed, helpless, hopeless, passive, anxious, guilt-ridden, isolated, defensive, confused, disorganized and self-deprecating. Any problem severe enough to bring a woman to a therapist might trigger these symptoms in a single-parent mother. By recognizing the external stress factors and the internal responses to them, a clinician can be of assistance to this woman. Without this acknowledgement, the clinician risks becoming a destructive agent, by intentionally or unintentionally blaming the victim of her plight. What follows is a basic model of a treatment plan for single-parent mothers who are having difficulty adjusting to the single-parent situation. Rather than assessing weaknesses, the plan is aimed at uncovering strengths.

Model

Generally the model will be completed in sequence, yet the stages are never fully completed nor isolated from each other. The specifics of the individual case must always be identified when attempting to apply the model. In addition, some clients may arrive in therapy having dealt with some of the issues previously. If the divorce or loss is far enough in the past, the issues surrounding it may have been resolved. The stress factors related to raising children single-handedly, though, may be complicating or aggravating other concerns. In other cases, single parents may be involved with or living with a partner who shares in child care, childrearing and the finances of the home. This may alleviate emotional and material burdens or in some cases create new ones.

The women with whom I am familiar do not always present themselves as victims of their circumstance. Some initiated divorce, some consciously chose to raise a child alone, and some are raising them with other partners, male or female. On the other hand, some are incest or rape victims, some were married and deserted and some were only eleven or fifteen when they chose to keep their baby. Despite the relative degree of happiness with their single parenthood status, financial burdens, stress and cultural socialization often may complicate their ability to provide the care, security and material goods the family needs. In all cases, though, it is important to remember that being a single-parent mother is not a clinical entity. It is a life circumstance that tends to be associated with various forms of stress.

It is important to distinguish between four female single-parent client situations: 1. One who is dealing or needs to deal with the emotional transition and the circumstances that led to single-parenthood, 2. One who is dealing with the stress of single-parenthood, 3. The client who has all the clinical symptoms of stress, disorganization, anxiety, feelings of being overwhelmed, but is unaware of the stress contributed by her single-parenthood status, 4. One who is a single parent, but whose own or family problems are basically unrelated to the circumstances of becoming or being a single-parent. By distinguishing these groups of clients, the model can be appropriately streamlined for each case. There is, of course, a fifth category, the single-parent mother who is managing her life satisfactorily and has no need for therapy. In this category are those who have been protected from the high levels of stress associated with single-parenthood via their ability to provide materially for their family, or via strong emotional and social support systems or those who can handle exceptionally well the high levels of stress associated with single-parenthood.

The model consists of six phases:

A. The establishment of trust and communication
B. The recognition of losses
C. The acknowledgement of single-parenthood
D. The identification of related stress factors
E. The development of skills and resources
F. The ability to separate and deal with unrelated issues.

A. Establishing Trust and Communication

Trust and communication between therapist and client must be established in order for the client to access therapy. Establishing trust and communication may be a monumental therapeutic task in and of itself. A number of client problems can interfere with the easy establishment of sufficient trust and communication to continue in the process of dealing with the problems of single-parenthood. These include: A client handicapped by severe difficulties in trusting others, or a client experiencing a psychotic episode, or a severe and incapacitating stress reaction or depression, alcoholism, defense mechanisms that prevent the client from attempting to seek help or a client who has difficulty overcoming the stigma of being "in therapy." These exemplify the variety of factors that prevent moving on to the next step. In the case of a single parent, a number of these difficulties may be a response to the overwhelming stress of single-parenting. A particularly relevant and often highly effective approach to overcoming trust difficulties in this population would be for the clinician to address the survival needs of the client directly and concretely. In the case of a sinking single parent, the clinician must meet survival needs by offering concrete relief either him/herself or via referral to an appropriate resource. Unless and until "real" survival needs are acknowledged and met by the clinician, the client will not be able to access her own inner resources in order to begin to address her own needs. Unless the survival needs are met, the woman will remain emotionally attached to a past source of emotional and material provisions and will remain unable to access her anger toward it. By substituting a new source of provisions the therapist will allow the client to become independent of the old one. Only then can the woman begin on the true road to independence. This leads us to the next stage.

B. *Recognizing Losses and the Selves Left Behind*

Along with dealing with the losses that have been incurred in cases of divorce, desertion, separation and death, other less apparent issues must be addressed. In order to overcome depression, these woman as well as the never-married woman, need to release their anger in many directions:

—at the father for the degree to which he escaped the concrete problems and societal judgements
—at society for putting her in a helpless position with inadequate material resources
—at herself for not being able to cope, even if the demands are superhuman
—at her guilt for not being able to provide as adequately for her children as she would like to do
—at society for making her feel less recognized as if she had lost status in society's eyes by becoming a single parent
—at the challenge to her belief that women and men are equal or that society or men take care of her when in fact she must support herself on 59 cents of each dollar a man earns.

Moving the depression toward anger and resolution will help the woman release energy to begin to build a new and stronger sense of self. Regardless of which partner initiated the leaving process, the woman will feel a great sense of relief when she is ready to move on from a situation that drained her energies rather than continued to support her.

C. *Acknowledging Single-Parenthood and Defining the Roles Involved*
and
D. *Identifying Stress Factors of Single Parenthood—Dealing With the Realities and the Emotional Responses*

These two categories will be discussed together as they occur to some degree simultaneously. At first they are approached by the clinician on an intellectual level, before they can be fully dealt with by the client on an emotional level. These two phases have the effect of helping the client define herself and the stress separately, thus allowing the client to step out of the problem and into a definition of herself. She begins with self-definition, self-organization and self-management, and these lead her to a more outer-directed problem definition, problem organization and problem management. By defining herself clearly she can define reality more clearly. She is no longer merged with the chaos of the problems, but instead has separated herself. Stress caused disorganization which in turn caused more stress. In analyzing intellectually and defining her emotional needs specifically, she has reduced her stress level and can now aim toward specific solutions.

E. Developing Skills and Resources

By offering the client specific skills, either formally or informally, the therapist has increased her effectiveness in the world and her self-esteem. These skills include: parenting skills, crisis prevention skills, home management skills, resource access skills, and networking and communication skills. The therapist must also aim to help the client find her own resolutions to the problems she has defined, whether they be material or interpersonal concerns. At this point the clinician can help the client see that her best functioning for herself and her children will come from increasing her use of appropriate support system—friends, relatives, and agencies. This will aid in alleviating her guilt which was motivated by her belief that she has to provide for her children single-handedly. It redefines her role as organizer and overseer of her own and her childrens' needs. She reestablishes her power (as opposed to her helplessness), and her capabilities, and directs her coping skills at organization and goal-oriented tasks. In this way, she minimizes her sense of being overwhelmed, incompetent and passive in the face of crises.

F. Dealing with Unrelated Issues

At this point the client is ready to deal with issues that are not directly related to being a single parent.

Guidelines

The following guidelines will be helpful to the therapist in working with this type of client: 1. The therapist must avoid being part of the problem. To do this she/he must not expect the impossible. 2. She/he must help the woman acknowledge the unfairness in appropriate cases, but simultaneously focus on the reality which must be faced. 3. She/he must acknowledge in the initial phases of therapy that the woman's own needs could not possibly be met, since the pressures on her are tremendous. Throughout the therapy the therapist should continue to identify actions which the woman takes to meet her own personal needs. 4. The therapist must make the woman cognizant of the fact that this is a crisis, not only of situation, but a crisis of roles, of trust of society, of adjustment to work, independent parenting, of loss of a spouse, and of whatever other factor arises for this woman. 5. The therapist needs to keep an updated list of appropriate resources for a parent in need.

Gains

In following the situational problem of single-parenting through these stages, the skills gained by the client in this sequence of development can be transferred to other areas. This gives the clinician and the client a solid basis for working on other issues. Some of the gains that can be observed will be new self-awareness, awareness of the environment and its impact on the individual client, new coping strategies, awareness of the ineffective use of defenses (e.g., denial), a more well developed and more accurate self-image, improved self-esteem, improved reality testing skills, organization and management skills to deal with self and the environment, and the experience of completing the emotional, intellectual and sequential work involved in problem-solving.

More basic issues are raised in this process and it is the therapists clinical judgement that determines to what extent these will be addressed while maintaining adherence to the format presented. The format calls for the client to leave therapy with a cognitive model for approaching problem-solving. This puts therapy in the context of self-empowering education, rather than in an authoritarian medical model which reinforces the dependence and the concept of flaw or illness in the patient.

In this model the client leaves with self-knowledge, skills, concrete evidence of progress and effectiveness and a view of herself as an actor in the environment. She also learns to see others as resources for support, knowledge and fulfillment of material needs.

Directions for Future Research

New research needs to be done to provide crucial information regarding needs and survival mechanisms for single parents. Research is needed that addresses child care, its availability, and the impact of its availability in increasing family income. Related factors would include researching the percentage of women single-parents with school-age children who are employed as compared to those with one or more children under six. What are the income levels of these two different household groups?

Research is needed that addresses job discrimination for women raising families. This would include comparing the income of single-parent males and females who have children under eighteen. If males generally earn twice as much as women under these circumstances, it would be interesting to compare the concomitant problems of individuals living at those median income levels regardless of sex. This would help determine what influences are purely income and lack of resource determined and which may be due to gender-related discrimination or socialization.

More extensive research must be done to determine whether males adjust to single-parenting more easily. Are they able to provide for more material needs, avoid more discrimination and do they have fewer role changes to make? Also, do males find it difficult to nurture children emotionally, and is this role lacking in single-parent male families? If so, what is the impact of these differences on the children? It would be important to use gender-related strengths to understand how to ameliorate the vulnerable areas in either gender's parenting.

Conclusion

Beyond the economic statistics, we have begun to explore the possible impact of discriminatory social policies, the effects of social mores and practices, discriminatory employment practices and access to community services, including child care on the single-parent, woman-headed family. Preliminary research suggests that these areas combine in an overwhelming fashion to produce mammoth stress factors for the single-parent mother. These stress factors are only further complicated by such factors as culturally-based socialization patterns for women and girls and attitudes and practices in traditional therapy. Under these combined conditions women often find it difficult to separate their own personal emotional problems from the external pressures and the crises that require immediate, practical solutions.

Alternative treatment strategies must include educating therapists and viewing therapy as in part an educational practice and a practice which provides concrete results for clients. In addition, the therapist may offer assertiveness training or support community networking to meet the family's survival needs in conjunction with therapeutic techniques. On a more indirect level, the therapist may attempt to change public or agency policy through research and pressure. Therapy, then, can be seen as a form of empowerment by providing the client with self-eduction in the form of therapy, awareness of external stress factors (including discriminatory attitudes and practices), skill training (e.g., in assertiveness or communication skills), emotional support, and protection in the form of client advocacy in the community.

REFERENCES

Newsweek, "Life Below the Poverty Line," New York: Vol. XCIX, No. 14, April 5, 1982.
US Department of Commerce Bureau of the Census, *Current Population Reports: Population Characteristics*, Series P-20 No. 324, "Population Profile of the United States: 1977," Issued April 1978.
US Department of Commerce Bureau of the Census, *Population Characteristics*, Series P-20 No. 307, "Households and Families by Type," Issued August 1978.

THE PSYCHOLOGICAL IMPACT OF FAMILY LAW ON DISPLACED HOMEMAKERS

Dorothy Dean McIntosh

The purpose of this study is to help to educate women and their children who may have been displaced through death, divorce, separation, desertion, or the disablement of their provider. A second, and equally important purpose is to help to educate all members of our society about the social and psychological impact of present family law policies and practices on women and children. As a participant observer who had once been displaced after 24 years as a homemaker, I am acquainted with some of the legal and psychosocial issues. As a clinician, I know that a large number of women are presently dealing with these issues, and therefore I am highly motivated to research the problems which need to be resolved. In-depth interviews with three women have been used to describe individual situations in vivo. The A.P.A. Ethical Principles in the Conduct of Research with Human Participants, 1973, have been used as a standard, and a statement of confidentiality was pledged to each participant. None of the subjects has been interested in notoriety or defaming the character of their husbands or former husbands.

In order to learn the history and background of family law which contributed to the present legal climate I reviewed the literature on the family, current findings, and historical trends. In general, there were four categories of literature:

a. Historical
b. Sociological
c. Psychological
d. Legal

It was also important to study the general conditions and prospects of women and their children who are struggling with this today. Legal resources were

---

Ms. McIntosh became a displaced homemaker at the age of 50. Her daughter died at the age of four, and she now has two grown sons. At the age of 54 she received a Master of Arts, and at 63 she is a doctoral candidate at Boston University. She is a Family Therapist.

obtained from a Professor of Family Law at Boston University Law School. Additional sources were obtained from *Ms Magazine*, the *Boston Globe*, professional journals, and other publications. Two pamphlets on women's economic contributions to the home and family were provided by one of the participants. Presentations at two professional women's conferences held in Boston during the spring of 1981 made valuable contributions to my study: the American Association of Women in Psychology Conference, and the National Conference on Women and the Law.

Family Law

At present, Family Law is undergoing reform, and is by no means uniform in every state (Family Law Reporter, 1980). The task of integrating the positive and negative aspects of this situation will require a long term research effort, due to differences of opinion on the issue of states' rights.

A good understanding of the historical background of English Common Law, as based upon the Judeo-Christian heritage of Christian Canon Law (Krause, 1976, pp. 127–129; Chafetz, 1974, pp. 139–140), may be summed up as follows:

> The state of the law described by Blackstone has been summarized to the effect that, under the common law, husband and wife were one person and that person was the husband. In the last century the so-called Married Women's Property Acts were enacted widely to improve the married woman's lot, indeed to provide equality between the spouses. In the current Canadian reform discussion (1975) . . . these laws have been criticized as a "theoretical concession to equality based upon nineteenth century laissez-faire economics" (Krause, p. 129).

According to Chafetz (1974) "with the exception of eight states (Arizona, California, Idaho, Louisiana, Nevada, New Mexico, Texas, and Washington) the legal system of our society is based directly on English Common Law; those eight are called community property states, and their legal system derives from Continental Europe. However, in practice, although not theory, their laws as they pertain to the subject at hand are quite similar in their effects to those of the other 42 states" (p. 139). The states are not united, however, in their individual handling of family and domestic relations, as these have been considered to be internal matters to be dealt with by each state.

The divisions between the states on the passage of the Equal Rights Amendment are illustrative of the difficulties in reaching a consensus

(Krause, 1976, pp. 289–291). Although this amendment has been introduced at every congressional session since 1923, and finally passed on March 22, 1972, the fate of the amendment is still uncertain; at this time three more states must ratify before June 30, 1982. In 1982 the controversy centers around the issues of protection and choice. Opponents of ERA use fear-producing tactics to cloud the issues and influence legislators. Although it is not true, for example, that states like Massachusetts which have their own Equal Rights Amendment have ceased to require that a husband must support his wife, or that women have been drafted, misleading statements which claim their concern to protect the rights of homemakers actually deny the double standard and sexual caste system which exists within the nuclear family (Chafetz, 1974, p. 141; Frieze, 1978, p. 300; Huber, 1973, pp. 52–54; Shields, 1980, pp. 130–133). In the meantime, much confusion and ignorance abounds, the victims of this condition often being the most confused and victimized (Goodman, 1981; Shields, 1980, pp. 5–10). Better knowledge of the law, more uniform laws, and revised legal ethics are imperative, in the opinion of the women I have interviewed. Rational thought, not emotional rhetoric, is needed. The president of the American Bar Association, David Brink, has stated that:

> The ERA will not affect private relations. It will not force women to enter the work force or interfere with whatever family structure may be established between husband and wife. It will protect homemakers by recognizing the dignity and economic contribution that a woman makes to her family, home and community (1982, p. 11).

Family law has been substantially influenced in the 1970s by the adoption of no-fault divorce laws in most states. This is one aspect of consensus which developed in response to greatly increased divorce rates in an unstable society. Since divorce statistics have increased over 5% since 1974, and the divorce rate among Americans over 45 has doubled in the last 20 years, "divorce law reform is desperately needed in behalf of women whose marriages of long duration are ending" (Shields, 1980, p. 214; Huffhines, 1981, p. 1).

Interviews with Displaced Homemakers

Client #1: Marjorie

We had been talking for about a half hour, and Marjorie was telling me about her 31 years of marriage to a successful doctor, now listed in Who's Who in America. Here are her words:

I had paid all the bills with my own money for fifteen years, and I really got tired of doing that, so I asked my husband to take over that responsibility. He had a good job teaching in a medical school, and we had had four children in seven years.

Anguish then welled up in her throat uncontrollably, she swallowed hard, and tears came to her eyes. She managed to say, with difficulty and with her face contorted in pain:

I went by myself to deliver each child. I had no help from him.

Only her iron-clad self-discipline, ingrained from years of mandatory self-control, kept her from letting go with a torrent of tears. After he gave the accounts to his secretary to pay, with his money, his secretary became his lover and they had an illegitimate child. The doctor was making a large salary (about $80,000 per year) but in the divorce settlement he forced his unemployed first wife of many years to repeatedly hire lawyers to defend herself and to regain the support money she had supplied while he was getting established in his profession. At the age of 60, Marjorie has earned a Masters degree and has opened a social service agency, trying to break even. Her children are all married and she lives alone.

In therapy, Marjorie would be helped to cry and express her feelings of anger, loss, and helplessness. A feminist approach would be supportive, provide assertiveness skills, referrals to competent feminist lawyers, and support groups made up of women with comparable intelligence and experience. Since Marjorie had above average resources of her own, she would be encouraged to take responsibility and find interests and satisfaction in helping other women, which she has done. She has also travelled and been encouraged to socialize. A regular evaluation of her progress in terms of self-image and future goals would be an integral part of the treatment program. The emphasis would be placed on re-building trust.

Client #2: Anne

Anne's hair, dark and waved, looked matted, as if she had been lying down before I arrived at her home. Her concern about her future was very evident. In an agitated tone she began her story.

I had to go into hiding with my young daughter so that her father could not kidnap her and take her out of the country with that other woman he was living with. We had to go on welfare, and he makes $100,000 a year. (He, too, is listed in Who's Who in America). I've had two lawyers and spent thousands of dollars on legal fees, but there's a double standard here. When he cohabits it is o.k., but I am isolated and alone, fighting for everything I get. I've felt so devastated that I burst into tears when a neighbor showed me kindness the other day.

Tears started falling down her cheeks in great drops as she wiped her face compulsively, and continued.

I feel demeaned and on the ragged edge, but he can travel, go to the ballet, and live in style. My daughter is never going to be foolish enough to go into marriage with her eyes closed, as I did.

A treatment plan for Anne would begin by working with her grief, her sense of loss and abandonment, and her anger. It would be supportive, building up her self-esteem and self-concept. (Although she had a Masters degree in Early Childhood Education, Anne had been unable to get a job. During a period of economic recession older women have difficulty competing with younger men and women for jobs). Assertiveness training skills are needed, as well as assistance in job searching. A referral network of competent feminist lawyers and a support group of other women would be incorporated in the treatment program. Since there is a high risk of depression, recreation and exercise as well as cognitive therapy are advised. A positive aspect of Anne's situation is the fact that she is needed by her young daughter who is still in school. A feminist therapist might want to invite the daughter to a few therapy sessions to help to re-inforce positive attitudes toward her mother. Goals of building trust, finding appropriate work, and improving Anne's self-image would be evaluated at least every month until marked improvement is evidenced. Her age is 45.

Client #3: Barbara

At 51, Barbara looked competent and self-controlled. She denied being a displaced homemaker, although she had been a house-spouse for 12 years.

I chose to divorce my husband because I was unhappy and bored. I had too much mental energy that was not being used. Since my parents were poor, and I had an older brother, the education money went to the male. I was expected to marry, and I did what I was expected to do. The romantic idea of marriage soon lost its appeal, as I was programmed to love marriage, not my husband. I felt trapped and unprepared to accept a life of routine housework, although I knew I could accomplish more. I requested no alimony, as I knew that money was my husband's security. He gave me minimum support for our two sons, and life has been painful for us financially.

After ten years of working at many uninteresting jobs, Barbara went back to college and has now completed her doctorate. She and her sons had no health insurance for years, and could not afford dental care. She says she prayed a lot and cried a lot, but feels she and her sons have a sense of bonding they would not have had otherwise. They all know they can survive on a minimum of money, and have no desire to exchange their life style for a plastic house like their father's and his trips to Europe. Barbara confessed that she invites no friends to her apartment because the furniture is so shabby. Nothing has been replaced, and if something breaks it is discarded.

Barbara looked rather sad when she said:

My mother has punished me by refusing to baby-sit when I needed help, and my brother won't speak to me. He has invited my mother to his house for Thanksgiving dinner, and I will be alone.

Wistfully, she smiled a sad smile, and said: "But I don't mind, it will be just like any other day off from work." She enjoys her work as a Family Therapist.

Although therapy was indicated for many years, Barbara has shown initiative and strength of self-concept by her independent decisions and courage to become responsible for herself and her two sons. Had she known what was ahead of her she might not have gone ahead, but she was young enough to work, and free enough to get by without material possessions. She did have the advantage of renting an apartment from her mother, which supplied her with some security. Feminist therapists and supportive networks have been available in the area where Barbara lives, and she has also relied on cultural and educational resources. Loneliness and pain have been overcome by hard work and perseverance. She enjoys helping others, and has succeeded at long last in actualizing her potential.

The psychological issues which have emerged to date are: intense pain, anger, shock, grief, insecurity, powerlessness, helplessness, frustration, loneliness, conflict, anxiety, incredulity, disgust, feelings of being demeaned unjustly, feelings of abandonment of children and spouse, low self-esteem, low self-concept, depression, and disillusionment. Social issues are: lack of equal protection under the law, economic insecurity and hardship, job discrimination, age discrimination, lower social status, inadequate health care, inadequate housing, and isolation. In families where this has not left bitterness, the security of the homemaker and her offspring has not been based on material conditions, but on hard work, willingness to do menial labor, sacrifice, and independent striving. In each family, it was felt that dependency was a high price to pay for the temporary security of a home and a provider.

Discussion

As we have seen, equality and equal protection under the law are a long way away, in spite of some cases decided in women's favor by the United States Supreme Court; i.e., the Equal Employment Opportunity Act of 1972, which is still being implemented (Faludi, 1981). An article on economic opportunity for women which appeared in the Boston Globe (Stocker, 1980) gave current figures "estimated by insurance companies on the market value of full-time homemaker's labor." The figure was then $16,000 per year. Studies on this subject have been going on since 1970 (Leghorn & Warrior, 1974), and an International Campaign for Wages for Housework has been organized for several years, without success to date. Yet, in the case of divorce, alimony "is usually for 1 to 2 years, if granted at all, and only 46% of the 14% who are awarded alimony receive it with any regularity" (Shields, 1980, p. 15). Child support is an equally frustrating problem, since most children live with their mothers at present, and support payments are often difficult to enforce (National Conference on Women and the Law, 1981). Many women do not realize, until too late, that only minor children are entitled to support of any kind. Even educational support is not guaranteed, and must be carefully negotiated. Many lawyers do not educate mothers about these loopholes, and the ignorance of a woman becomes the escape clause for a man who lacks a sense of responsibility toward his children.

L. S., a widow, found that she could not get a job due to age discrimination. She was 54. Pension rights and Social Security inequities are both in need of reform. A series of articles on Women in Poverty by the *Boston Globe* confirmed the predicament of economic insecurity which plagues the displaced homemaker (Dumanoski, 1980). The feminization of poverty has been demonstrated by recent studies: 30% of female-headed households are below the poverty line, and these comprise 51% of all those below the poverty line (Levitan and Belous, 1981, p. 22).

Implications of Study

We find that the psycho-social issues which have emerged from the interviews are generally in line with the literature on sex roles. According to Frieze (1978), women have had to live with de facto discrimination for ages:

> Throughout history, women have had fewer rights and lower social status than men. This inequity has led to a number of negative consequences for women: economic hardship; loss of self-esteem; feelings of powerlessness; lowered control over external events; etc. It is not difficult to see that social and economic discrimination can make women's lives more difficult (p. 270).

The women whom I have interviewed were all intelligent, highly educated women who felt demeaned by being devalued as persons. When two of these women had to fight their wealthy husbands to protect themselves and their children after ten to thirty years of domestic service, insult was added to injury.Ironically, the displaced homemaker is invariably the woman whose high ideals took precedence over her own economic security, and who conscientiously devoted her most productive years to the up-bringing of her children as well as the career aspirations of her husband. Her anger and disillusionment as well as depression, are appropriate responses to the devaluing of her contributions to the welfare of her family. As Gilligan (1981) has pointed out: "Women start with a premise of connection. The pronoun *we* predominates. Women don't break early ties and add relationships, but ask how they can sustain the connection" (AWP Conference, 1981).

REFERENCES

Black, H. C. *Black's law dictionary*. St. Paul: West, 1979.
Blackstone, W. *Commentaries on the laws of England*. Oxford: Clarendon Press, 1765.
Bonavich, P. Allocation of private pension benefits as property in Illinois divorce proceedings. *DePaul Law Review*, Fall, 1979, 29:1–46.
Brink, D. Debate exaggerates ERA impact. *National NOW Times*, April, 1982, 15: #3, p. 11.
Chafetz, J. S. *Masculine, feminine, or human*? Illinois, Peacock Publishers, Inc., 1974, 1978.
Dover, A. P. Financial equality in marriage and parenthood. *Catholic University Law Review*, Spr. 1980, *29*: 733–750.
Dumanoski, D. The new poor: women, children. *Boston Globe*, December 14, 1980, 218: #167.
Faludi, S. Harvard will reopen woman's tenure case. *Boston Globe*, April 12, 1981, pp. 21 & 26.
Family law reporter, Bureau of National Affairs, Washington, D. C., 1980 supplements.
Fishman, C. Phyllis Schlafly. The liberated anti-feminist explains her world view. *The Harvard Independent*, April 16, 1981, pp. 13–14.

Frieze, I. H., Parsons, J. E., Johnson, P. B., Ruble, D. N., & Zellman, G. L. *Women and sex roles.* New York: W. W. Norton & Co., 1978.

Gatto, P. Women share ideas, concerns at law conference. *Boston Globe,* April 5, 1981, p. 26.

Gilligan, C. Woman's place in man's life cycle. *Harvard Educational Review,* November 1979, *49*: #4.

Gilligan, C. Women's moral development and psychological theory. Presentation at *AWP National Conference,* Boston, Massachusetts, March, 1981.

Gilligan, C. *In a different voice.* Cambridge, Harvard University Press, 1982.

Glendon, M. A. Modern marriage law and its underlying assumptions: The new marriage and the new property. *Family Law Quarterly,* Winter, 1980, *13*: 441-460.

Goldstein, J. E. Children born of marriage. *Mo. Law Review,* Spring, 1980, *45*: 307-16.

Goodman, E. Women and children last. *Washington Post,* March 14, 1981.

Hebert, C. S. Enforcement of contractual separation agreements by specific performance. *Wake Forest Law Review,* Fall, 1980, *16*: 117-36.

Huber, J. Ed. *Changing women in a changing society.* Chicago, University of Chicago Press, 1973.

Huffhines, K. Women over 40 and alone. *The Brookline Tab,* April 15, 1981, p. 1.

Jacobs, R. H. *Life after youth: female, forty—what next?* Boston: Beacon Press, 1979.

Krause, H. D. *Family law, cases and materials.* St. Paul: West, 1976.

Leghorn, L. & Warrior, B. *What's a wife worth?* Boston: N. E. Free Press, 1974.

Levitan, S. A. & Belous, R. B. *What's happening to the American family?* Baltimore: Johns Hopkins University Press, 1981.

Miller, J. B. *Toward a new psychology of women.* Boston: Beacon Press, 1975.

National Conference of Women and the Law. Women and justice: blind no more. Boston: April, 1981.

Newhall, G. *Settlement of estates and fiduciary law in Massachusetts.* Rochester, N. Y.: Lawyer's Co-operative Publishing Co., 1958.

Rheinstein, M. *Marriage stability, divorce, and the law.* Chicago: University of Chicago Press, 1972.

Rosen, M. Dehumanizing effects of sex stereotypes. *Psychiatric Opinion,* February, 1978, p. 28.

Rothman, S. *Woman's proper place.* New York: Basic Books, 1978.

Russell, L. *Growth in partnership.* Philadelphia: Westminster Press, 1981.

Schlafly, P. The case against the ERA. *Radcliffe Quarterly, March, 1982, 68*: #1.

Shields, L. *Displaced homemakers, organizing for a new life.* New York: McGraw-Hill, 1980.

Stocker, C. The picture is gloomy for women in the 80s. *Boston Globe,* November 23, 1980.

THE BLACK SISTERHOOD:
A SECOND LOOK

Helen Boulware Moore

Introduction

Supermamas, Matriarchs, Two-for-oners: names which have been used
to characterize contemporary black women, each implying that they possess
"something special" that makes them different from their black mates and
from both white males and white females. in fact, this "something special"
which has made black women different and has influenced their behavior
in the United States is the double dose of discrimination, the powerful hands
of racism and sexism, the "double whammy." Unlike their black mates,
black women have not been included in the male chauvinistic Ole Boy Network. Unlike their white female counterparts, black women have not been
invited into the exclusive "white only" club. Unlike white males, black
females have little power. Both the Black Power and the Women's
Movements held out promises of entry into the mainstream of American life
to black women, but in many ways, the promises have been hollow and
empty.

A look at the statistics reported by the United States Department of Commerce, Bureau of Census, 1973, indicates that about one half (48.6%) of
black women in this country over the age of sixteen were involved in the
civilian work force as compared with approximately 44.6% of their white
counterparts. This figure changed in 1978 to 48.5% of white females and
53.3% of black females and rose again in 1979 to 50.6% of white females
and 53.5% of black females who were involved in the civilian work force
(Handbook of Labor Statistics, December 1980). Differences in work participation between black and white women were a function of the woman's
marital status and her race. The presence of young children in the home affected the work status of black women less than it did white women in the
same category. Among women with children over the ages of five years,

Helen Boulware Moore is the Director of Supportive Instructional Services at Simmons
College. Additionally, she is a member of the psychology department where she teaches a
psychology of women course. Dr. Moore is a licensed psychologist specializing in the psychology
of women.

larger proportions of black women as compared with white women were active in the labor force (Handbook of Labor Statistics, December 1980).

In and of itself, these statistics sound like good news. Black women were being employed in the civilian work force in increasing numbers as promised by both the Black Power and the Women's Movements. However, the other side of the statistical story indicates that the news may not be so good after all. In 1979 12.3% of black women over the age of sixteen were unemployed as compared with a figure of 5.9% of white women in the same category. Additionally, black working women were clustered in the craftsmen and service jobs with 50.3% of black working women as compared with 33.6% of working white women being employed as skilled laborers and service workers. At the managerial level, 3.4% of black women were employed as managers while 6.8% of white women and 6.9% of black men were managing. 14.9% of white males were managers. At the professional level, white women were employed at the rate of 16.4% to 14.2% of black women. The statistics cited above demonstrate that while black women were entering the civilian work force in increasing numbers, their rise to higher levels of white collar professions has been slow and hesitating. Black women represent a very small group at the middle managerial level; they are virtually absent in senior level management (Handbook of Labor Statistics, December 1980).

The reality of the statistics from the United States Department of Labor draws a striking contrast with the prevailing perceptions of black women. How does it happen that so many so-called "Supermamas" and "Matriarchs" (50.3% of employed black women) find themselves at the lower end of the employment scale? Why have not more employers, in pursuit of affirmative action brownie points, hired black women who would satisfy both racial and sexual guidelines? Racism and sexism have combined to form a "double whammy" in the employment picture of black women in this country.

Psycho-Social History of Black Women in America

The role of black slave women gives us an initial clue to the interaction of history and the present-day psyches of contemporary black females. The activities of the slave women in the homes and lives of the slave masters and their families put them in an optimal position to become familiar with the operations of the dominant culture. Not only were slave women required to do the masters' bidding in their kitchens and their laundries, but they were also forced into servitude in the bedrooms, often listening to their inner thoughts and dreams, activities usually reserved for husband/wife relationships. Their freedom to move in and out of the white world was not abandoned with the Emancipation Proclamation. During the one hundred years of hard struggles between 1865 and 1965, black women had greater knowledge of and were less of a threat to the dominant white culture than were their black mates. It was they who could be hired in the white kitchens when jobs were difficult to find for black males. Black females have been able to exist in close liaison with white America, and consequently, have knowledge of both cultures, black and white.

American society has traditionally placed the physical attributes of white females on a pinnacle. For this culture, white skin, long blond hair, and keenness of features were considered determinants of femininity. Black women did not possess any of these characteristics claimed by white society to be the essence of beauty. In a real sense, society was denying black women their claim to femininity. The setting of physical standards by white society that excluded black females from participation in American standards of beauty also had its effects on the psyches of black women. To this reality, according to noted black psychiatrists, Grier and Cobbs, black women responded with a shift from traditionally developed narcissism, love of self, to a non-traditional narcissistic interest in achievement, indications of an inner beauty. What can we do to prove our self-worth, they asked? Black women did not concern themselves with femininity in the traditional sense and were thus less affected by societal restrictions placed on servitude to feminine roles. They were freed of the restraints binding white females. So while the non-traditional development of narcissism has served to protect black women from the pangs of rejection, it has also served to remove from them the demands of societal obedience to sex appropriate roles (Grier and Cobbs, 1968). Black women were free to reach out to each other and to their communities, to take roles of leadership and support both in their homes and in their work places.

Kardiner and Ovesey (1971) in *The Mark Of Oppression* point out that while the aspirations and drives to achieve of blacks are often high, social barriers are such that symbolic substitutions of goals are frequently necessary. Thus black women, in the face of near impossible movement up the social and economic ladder, were forced to replace their original goals of high professional achievement with substitute goals. Grier and Cobbs have suggested that such substitutions may have been centered around black women's direction of energies into nurturing. Black women were supportive of each other not only within the nuclear family but extending to the community and church family as well. It was not an uncommon sight to see neighbors caring for each other's young or to hear one black sister speaking to her boss on behalf of another. The black community thrived on the love and attention of devoted "aunts" who shared no blood relationship with their nieces and nephews. Mama in *A Raisin in the Sun* is a familiar face within the traditional black community, and her exalted presence goes back to the black woman's ancestry on the African continent. In deflection of other directed energies, traditional black women guarded their brood against the evils of the outside world and directed their ambitions toward that which was uniquely theirs, nurturance.

With the rise of the Black Power movement in the mid to late sixties, black females found themselves at the center of a cultural renaissance. Blacks as a group were experiencing a "death of the defense posture," a reordering of approaches to the old problem of the black experience in America. No longer was it necessary for the black mother to defend her family from racist hostility in the same way. Laws that protected blacks from racial abuse were passed and began to be enforced. The black movement was forcing the issue of acceptance of blacks as they were, not as whites would have liked them to be. Blacks felt freer to be competent, assertive, and vocal in issues regarding their life affairs. Aunt Jemina was dying (Jeffers, 1970).

There was an acknowledgment that "black is indeed beautiful" and the recognition of black females as true objects of beauty. Large cosmetic firms clamored for their business, and department store counters, once filled with "white only" potions, catered also to the sepia-toned. The advent of the mini-skirt in the late sixties proved to America that the long, tapered legs of the ebony model were stylish and chic. The Afro hair style flourished, allowing black women to thrive in natural radiance without an obligation to mimic white styles. All of this made a positive statement to the once divested narcissistic system of black females. Black women began to see themselves in significant numbers as models in fashion magazines and actresses on stage, screen, and television. Black women in this country began to move out of the laundries and kitchens and into the professional world. No longer was entrance into public life guarded by physical likeness to white standards of beauty. Top fashion models like Naomi Sims and actress Cicely Tyson, representatives of African beauty standards, signified to black women that their physical attributes were relevant to America's new expanding standards of beauty.

The passage of civil rights acts and laws governing equal employment opened the doors of opportunity for black women. Both the Women's Movement and the Black Movement were saying to black females, "Opportunity is yours. Step out and take it." Within the black movement, black women were beginning to reassess themselves in light of new evidence. No longer were black women filled with guilt for crimes of rape and sexual abuse thrust upon them during slavery. The reassessment of their self-images made way for new and exciting adventures.

While only a few years ago black women thought of themselves as Negro, at the end of the Black Power movement, African-American women spoke of themselves as Black. "One of the most powerful goals of the Black Power revolution was to make mainstream life rewards within the grasp of the average black individual. Whether the black revolutionary sought black-instigated apartheid, or merely a more powerful voice in black-related affairs, the fundamental goals were not too different from what one might consider mainstream American life goals: feelings of pride in self and group, security for self and family, self-enhancing work and leisure activities, freedom from hunger, violence, illness, and control over one's destiny" (Bank and Grambs, 1972, p. 274). Thus contemporary black women saw the vision of moving out of the kitchen and into the board room, a vision of finding relief from the heavy burden that had been their lot for centuries, a vision of expressing their truly feminine nature, and a vision of having options. For after all, wasn't the battle just about over? Hadn't they, like their black mates, been promised that a new day had dawned? Isn't America the land of the free and the home of the brave? But, America played a cruel trick on black women. Black power gains have been short lived, and life has called black women back to business as usual. They are left with feelings of frustration, anger, and despair. Affirmative Action is not working. They are still at the bottom of the economics totem pole. The doors to the board room have not opened for them. Their lot has not changed very much.

The responses of black women to their experience of double oppression are as varied as are the women themselves who comprise the group. The black experience in America has not been a monolithic one, and variations on the theme must be noted. Traditionally when faced with threats, many black women have responded by seeking safety within the group, reaching out for comfort, security, and nurturance from other groups members. Others have reached deep within themselves for intestinal fortitude to see themselves through difficult times. These women have tended to function within the presence of the group but not relying on the group for security. Others, however, have chosen to fulfill their safety needs by identifying with the aggressors, taking on the points of view of those who have chosen to oppress them. This syndrome is not peculiar to black women, and it has been documented as a defense mechanism used by members of a number of oppressed groups. Some of the Jews who were subjected to the holocaust in Germany and some of the white women involved in the Women's Movement are only two such examples. The term "trashing" has been used to label this behavior by the Women's Movement. These black women, each one in her own way, have become "the company women," making a decision to pull away from the group and thus isolating themselves from their natural source of support and nurturance. The unconscious motive that is operational with this group of women is the hope that they will somehow be viewed as different from the total group, thus making themselves less vulnerable to the "double whammy." The nature of racism and sexism in this country has not been selective, however, thus leading to anger and frustration as these black women face the reality of their oppression. They feel helpless and hopeless when weighing the alternatives in their lives, and they lash out at those whom they consider to be safe targets. Their displaced anger serves as the stimulus for black on black emotional violence as they express their competitiveness and aggression toward their black sisters. America has shown them that it is dangerous to express rage at the true oppressors; their needs for safety still their hands and quiet their voices. So they turn against their own and attack those who are a part of themselves. It is this final group of women about whom the remainder of the paper is concerned.

Clinical Case Material

Abraham Maslow's Hierarchy of Needs provides a theoretical framework with which to view the clinical case material which exemplifies the defiant behavior that is the response of some black women to what they perceive as their plight in America today. Maslow builds his hierarchy on the assumption that all human needs are not of equal potency, namely that the primary needs are of biological and physiological functioning—hunger, thirst, sex, elimination, etc. Of secondary importance is the need for safety, followed by the need for love, the need for self-esteem, and the need for psychological health and growth which Maslow terms the need for self-actualization (Coleman, 1976). "According to Maslow, needs on the lower levels are prepotent as long as they are unsatisfied. When they are adequately satisfied, however, the 'higher' needs occupy the individual's attention and effort" (Coleman, 1976, p. 107).

Given Maslow's analysis of needs and the prepotent relationship between lower level needs and needs which are nearer the top of the hierarchy, clinical case material suggests that the secondary need, the need for safety is being triggered in black American women by the influence of the "double whammy." Racism and sexism have created an atmosphere which is threatening to black women. They are isolated, lack financial and political parity with men of all races and with white women, find upward job mobility blocked, and are insecure about being taken seriously as professionals and as women. Black females are over-represented in the laborer and service categories (50.3%) but under-represented in professional and managerial jobs (17.6%) as compared with their white counterparts (23.2%). The discrepancy is equally as broad at the semi-professional and clerical levels where only 32.1% of black women as compared with 43.3% of white women are employed. Society has delivered the message to black women that jobs are not only scarce for them (unemployment rate of 12.3%), but, job advancement is difficult, if they are employed at all (Handbook of Labor Statistic, December 1980). Entry into upper level occupations by black women remain as tokenism only. Black women are not able to see themselves represented among those who have been employed in upper level jobs before them and some black women respond with fear to the professional implications of opening the doors for others to follow behind them. In this way some black women perpetuate the sense of isolation, the feelings of competition, and the tendency to pull away from professional encounters which require a spirit of cooperation and nurturant giving of themselves to others. An atmosphere of distrust and depression prevail, and their images of self are damaged. There is a need to rebuild the sisterhood.

CASE STUDY #1

Setting: Jane applied for a position as consulting psychologist in a large corporate plant. Her credentials included a PhD with 5 years of counseling experience. She was, however, unlicensed in the state at the time of application, although she was preparing for licensure. The job requirements were consistent with the skills that Jane had gained through her counseling experience and a state license was not required.

Situation: Jane had a sucessful first interview with the Personnel Manager who had been very open with his approval of her. He further indicated his desire to have Jane meet with the Plant Manager and look over the prospectus for the psychological services at the plant. Mary, a licensed black psychologist, had been hired to develop the O.D. program for the plant. Since she, too, was in the field of psychology, the Personnel Manager used her as a resource to review Jane's credentials. Without having an interview with Jane, Mary strongly suggested to the Personnel Manager that Jane not be hired for the position because she was not as yet licensed.

Results: 1. Mary was Queen Bee, the only black female psychologist at the plant site.
             2. The consultant's position was filled by a white male psychologist.
             3. Jane found out that her credentials were judged unfairly without a chance to respond.
             4. Jane felt bitter, angry, and unreceptive to collegiality with other black women in her field.

CASE STUDY #2

Setting: Black women's social service organization composed of professional black women representing a variety of professions and academic disciplines.

Situation: The club has agreed to work on a service project requiring expertise in the area of negotiations of contracts. One of the club members, Jane, is a lawyer skilled in this area. Jane has offered to negotiate the contracts for the project committee, indicating to the committee her sensitivity to their needs to keep the costs down while maximizing the efficacy of the project. Without deliberation, Jane's offer was flatly refused by the project committee with the additional insinuation that her offer was somehow self-serving in its intent.

Results: 1. The organization paid 20 to 25% more for the services than they might have paid had the contracts been negotiated by a skilled negotiator.
             2. The committee members felt hostile to the offer for assistance, preferring to inflate the project budget in lieu of allowing Jane to assist them.
             3. Jane is left feeling brushed off, isolated, and hurt by the committee's rejection. It is unlikely that she will reach out again to offer her expertise to the group.
             4. The organization has lost a valuable resource.

CASE STUDY #3

Setting: Jane had recently opened a beauty salon in a suburban community. She rented a salon in a building that housed several other office suites. Mary, an unlicensed beautician apprentice, aproached Jane asking for a job, indicating that she had trained at a white cosmetology school and that she desired to learn more about black hair care. Jane hired Mary, and during the next year, gave her a considerable amount of time and instruction. Mary's skills improved greatly.

Situation: Jane had a disagreement with the landlord and agreed to move. The arrangement called for a grace period of six months during which time Jane was to search for a new salon location and the landlord was to find a new tenant. Mary, who was still working with Jane at the time, contacted the landlord and expressed her interest in opening a salon of her own with an immediate occupancy date. The landlord saw an opportunity to effect a quick solution to his rental problems and gave Jane a one week eviction notice.

Results:
1. Jane lost her salon and had to go to work with another beautician in a nearby salon.
2. Mary, who was still unlicensed, opened a new salon in violation of the state code.
3. Jane felt hurt and betrayed by Mary whom she had helped.
4. Mary lost customers because of her deceit.

Intervention

The examples cited above point to the conflict that exists between the importance to the group of the traditional expression of nurturance by black women in America and the sense of competition with the group that some black women feel, especially in the marketplace. What happens when this group of black women embraces two conflicting cognitive elements in this way? In a study of attitudes and attitude change, Leon Festinger investigated "the relations among 'cognitive elements' and the consequences when the elements are inconsistent with one another" (Kiesler et al., 1969, p. 191). Cognitive elements are defined as bits of knowledge or opinions, beliefs about oneself, about one's behavior, and about one's surroundings in the environment. These two cognitive elements may be: traditional black women's nurturance served as one of the key ingredients in the survival of their people, and some contemporary black women have turned away from nurturance and have become competitive with their black sisters.

Using Festinger's theory, there can be three possible results. The cognitive elements may have no relationship whatsoever: traditional black women's nurturance served as one of the key ingredients in the survival of their people, and contemporary black women outnumber their black mates in this country. Or the relationship between elements may be compatible: traditional black women's nurturance served as one of the key ingredients in the survival of their people, and contemporary black women are nurturant to their sisters and brothers. Or the relationship between cognitive elements may be dissonant: traditional black woman's nurturance served as one of the key ingredients in the survival of their people, and some contemporary black women have turned away from nurturance and have become competitive with their black sisters.

Festinger suggests that "the existence of dissonance creates psychological tension or discomfort and will motivate the person to reduce the dissonance and achieve consonance" (Kiesler et al., 1969, p. 134–194). When cognitive dissonance exists, the person will be moved to change the precipitating attitude or behavior so as to reduce the inner-conflict that exists, thus achieving equilibrium or consonance. "When dissonance exists, not only will the person attempt to reduce it, but (s)he will actively attempt to avoid situations and information which would increase the dissonance" (Kiesler et al., 1969, p. 194). Thus black women confronted with cognitive dissonance will either change the opinions and behavior to reduce the dissonance or avoid situations and information which point up the dissonance. In other words, they will deny and run away!

Three strategies for intervention are appropriate as therapuetic treatment for the problems described above. The therapy group, limited to six clients, is designed for those women whose behavior is least adaptive to their interpersonal environment. The manifest affect is depression with accompanying anxiety. Each client is interviewed individually for a minimum of three treatment sessions to assess case history and to ascertain appropriate placement within the therapy group. Each client is assisted in setting therapy goals for treatment and to contract work toward these goals with the therapist and the group. The support group, limited to ten participants, is designed for those who feel the need now to reach out to others, who are similar to themselves, for feedback and support during crisis. The manifest affect is anxiety with intermittent depression. Candidates for the support group are coping moderately well to well in their interpersonal environments, although they sometimes feel anxious about the efficacy of their coping skills. Each client is interviewed individually for the initial treatment session to ascertain levels of anxiety and the appropriateness of placement in the support group. Support group members contract with each other and with the therapist to share their feelings and give feedback openly and honestly. Both the therapy and the support groups meet for 1½ hours weekly. The third intervention strategy is a professional network which is open to as many clients as are interested. Sessions are held only once a month for 1½ hours, and clients are free to attend on a regular or a periodic basis. The network is designed for women whose experiences on their jobs are less than satisfactory and who are seeking change. The network format includes group discussion on topics of professional interest led by the therapist or a guest speaker, sharing of both leads and needs for job change, and the development of contacts for job advancement. The network is appropriate for black women who are coping adequately, experiencing a minimal degree of concern about their job performance, and is open to all black women who wish to participate.

The choice of group therapy, support group, or black women's professional network depends on the actual circumstances of each client's case, the length and severity of her depression, as well as the nature of maladaptive behavior that is manifest as a response to the environment. All three strategies use group modality and cognitive therapy as a theoretical orientation. Cognitive therapy is "based on an underlying theoretical rationale that an individual's affect and behavior are largely determined by the way in which (s)he structures the world. Her cognitions are based on attitudes or assumptions. . .developed from previous experience" (Beck et al., 1981, p. 3). The therapeutic technique helps the client separate reality from distortion thus correcting the dysfunctional beliefs that underldy the cognitions (Beck, 1981). A variety of cognitive and behavioral tools are used in cognitive therapy. Manipulation of cognitive dissonance serves as the primary tool in the three intervention strategies described above.

The problems which bring clients into treatment relate to interpersonal issues which have shaped their opinions about the group. A group format has been chosen, therefore, as an appropriate modality for intervention. Within the safety of the group and in the presence of evaluative feedback from both the therapist and other group members, the client is encouraged to work on issues of self-image and trust. Feedback from the group assists the client in assessing her personal qualities, attributes, and opinions in light of the impact of racism and sexism on the reality of her life. The group setting simulated the real life existence which has caused stress in her life, and the client seeks to develop coping strategies to lessen the impact of the "double whammy." In this manner, the group helps the individual develop new, more adaptive patterns of behavioral response.

BIBLIOGRAPHY

Banks, James A. and Grambs, Jean D. *Black Self-Concept*. New York, NY: Harper and Row, 1972.
Beck, Aaron T. et al. *Cognitive Therapy of Depression*. New York, NY: The Guilford Press, 1981.
Coleman, James C. *Abnormal Psychology and Modern Life, 5th Edition*. Glenview, Ill: Scott Foresman and Company, 1976.
Grier, William H. and Cobbs, Price M. *Black Rage*. New York, NY: Basic Books, Inc., 1968.
Handbook of Labor Statistics, United States Department of Labor, Bureau of Labor Statistics. Washington, DC: December 1980.
Jeffers, Lance. "The Death of the Defensive Posture: Toward Grandeur in Afro-American Letters." *The Black 70's*. Edited by Floyd Barbour. Boston, MA: Porter Sargent Publishers, Inc., 1970.
Kardiner, Abram and Ovesey, Lionel. *The Mark of Oppression*. New York, NY: Norton Press, 1971.
Kiesler, Charles A. et al. *Attitude Change, A Critical Analysis of Theoretical Approaches*. New York, NY: Wiley and Sons, Inc., 1969.
United States Bureau of the Census, Current Population Reports. Special Studies, series p-23, No. 48. "The Social and Economic Status of the Black population in the United States, 1973." Washington, DC: 1974.

WOMEN'S CAREER DECISION-MAKING PROCESS: A FEMINIST PERSPECTIVE

Gail Washor-Liebhaber

"Work can be a way for individuals to express their identity and to explore their potential for competency and self-actualization. Women, however, seem unable to make choices about work in their lives." (Harmon, 1978) As a career counselor, I have found this grim observation to be all too true of the women who have come to consult with me over the past few years. They feel overwhelmed by the obstacles that they are just beginning to recognize and face. Anger, fear, anxiety, confusion—these are only a few of the feelings that suddenly come alive when women begin to ask themselves that age-old question: What do I want to be?

Whereas men are taught from the time that they are toddlers that they will work and be productive, women have received ambivalent messages about their vocational futures. Some of the luckier ones, with the support of parents, friends, peers, make good decisions and pursue their potential in the world of work. Others drift, wait, or settle for less. Many others still find themselves asking the question that once was a challenge and is now a threat. But if they look deeper they find that this question is not simply a matter of deciding *what* they want to be but *if* they want to be.

These women are creating options where before none existed. They are confronting issues of competency and skill level, of decision-making and risk-taking, and the very basic issues of self-confidence and esteem. For many the questioning goes deeper. They stand on the slippery edge of discovering that they are missing something in life—a sense of purpose, of direction. They are questioning their very identity.

Why do women have this struggle? And perhaps even more importantly, how can women respect their own vocational developmental process and learn to use it to help them grow? These and other questions will be answered by my experiences both personally and professionally as a career counselor.

Gail Washor-Liebhaber is a career counselor in private practice in Cambridge, MA. She specializes in facilitating groups for women and counseling adolescents. This article is an adaptation of the manual "Career/Life Issues: A Women's Support Group."

51

Career Development Theory and Women

Although career development theory is a relatively young science (the pioneering research which is still used today is less than thirty years old), it reflects a traditional view of women's place in the working world. In fact, aside from a few notable exceptions, researchers seem to suggest by their research methods that women have no place at all. The major contributors— Super, Roe, Holland, Ginzberg, Tiedman—all used male samples and norms when developing their particular brand of career development theory. When and if they considered women at all, which Super and Holland did in later studies, they succeeded in raising more questions than they could answer.

During the past seven years more and more women are conducting the research and so these questions are beginning to be answered in earnest. There was, however, one woman who was a contemporary of the above mentioned theorists who conducted an insightful study in 1964.

In a cross-cultural study, Tyler and her associates questioned school age boys and girls in the Netherlands and the Mid-West. The following remarks were in the closing paragraphs:

> It also seems likely that girls in the U.S. because of their over-riding importance to them of demonstrating their femininity are somewhat less free than girls in the Netherlands to develop their own individuality. The many specific sex differences we picked up in our study call for little special comment because they are so much in line with the prevailing opinion about how boys and girls differ. But the fact that. . . indices were so high for as to place all but one of the girls in one big cluster may lead to the questions of whether girls' attitudes are too stereotypical, too standardized. Many persons and agencies have recently become concerned about the failure of American females to make full use of their potentials.

Tyler goes on to state what she believes to be some of the causes of this condition:

> Inferior planning resting on too restricted a concept of femininity may be an important source of these difficulties. The fact that Dutch girls do not differ so much from boys suggests that something about our social norms rather than something inherent in human nature is involved here.

Since Tyler's research many social scientists, psychologists and researchers (mostly women) have documented how sex role socialization with its stereotypical expectations and beliefs influence the growth of our children. Career choices, or the seeming lack thereof, is just one arena where both males and females are affected in a negative way. For males, the expectation is that they will grow up to be task-oriented, competitive, productive, i.e., "work hard and the world is yours." Unfortunately, the roles of husband and father with the attendant characteristics of valuing home, family, and emotional growth are seen as secondary. Girls typically grow up envisioning their role in life in terms of affiliation, emotional security and pleasing/helping others.

Who are women trying to be and who are they attempting to please? According to a recent Gallup poll, 94% of all women still consider marriage to be the most satisfying way of life. Women are clearly valuing relationships over achievements. Jean Baker Miller has explored how and why women develop such strong affiliation needs in her book, *Towards a New Psychology of Women*. Dr. Miller emphasized that these emotional needs are implanted in a girl at the time that she is born by the way she is talked to, taught, played with, and perceived. It is by being kind, loving and nice that females are recognized and rewarded in her daily life. She learns at a young age that being alone (that is, without a man) is not to have any meaning in life.

Karen Horney summed it up this way in 1932: "women are, while...men do...female identity is ascribed, masculine identity achieved...she performs her part by merely being...the man on the other hand, has to do something to fulfill himself."

Growing Up Female—Factors of Career Choice

The process of career choice has been the subject of a great deal of research in the past ten years. As in most forms of socialization there are a few factors which are most easily identified as important influencers. Various family situations, peers, teachers, mentors, social and economic class, geographic location have all been analyzed.

The role of the mother has been found to be extremely important. The attitudes that the mother holds about employment are especially significant for girls, and if the mother herself is employed, her employment apparently affects the career behaviors and attitudes of both her sons and daughters.

The role of the mother also influences how her daughters perceive other women (and thus themselves) in a more general way.

Daughters of working mothers describe women as more competent and

effective than do daughters of non-working mothers. . . Hoffman and
Nye (1974) also found that college women who are career-oriented
or planning less conventionally feminine careers are likely to be
daughters of working mothers, and there is some evidence that the
daughters of working mothers are more independent than daughters
of non-working mothers.

Investigation of the father's role suggests that his influence may be even
more powerful. Weitzman (1975) speculates that "an especially strong
stimulus for achievement motivation in women is a strong father-daughter
relationship in which the father makes his love and approval dependent upon
her performance rather than showing unconditional support whether or not
his daughter achieves."

Another factor worth discussing is the perceived attitude of significant
men in a female's adolescence and adulthood. As young girls we learn to
act according to expectations from others. In school we may try not to be
smarter, more athletic or funnier than the boys who we want to ask us to
go to the movies. We learn at a very young age about the not so mythical
male ego. As we get older our issues may change but our fears about acceptance and approval don't.

Matina Horner, famous for her research into the fear of success syndrome,
takes this idea one step farther: "It is especially difficult for a capable,
achievement oriented young woman whose sense of self-esteem includes feelings of competence or a desire for success in non-traditional areas to maintain any stable sense of identity or self-regard as a feminine woman."

In 1981 I was quite anxious to do some of my own research on girls who
might have working mothers and who might also be influenced by the more
liberating politics of a northeastern college town. Working as a career
counselor in a high school in Cambridge, Massachusetts provided me with
the opportunity of discovering first hand what some of the young women
were considering for their vocational futures. I developed a program to introduce the juniors and seniors to non-traditional jobs, which I defined as
anything other than secretarial, teaching or pink collar jobs. My attempts
were poorly received by the majority of girls who I saw. They were mostly
interested in the field of education despite a well-known state-wide cut-back
in the hiring of teachers. I was shocked to find most assuming that they would
get married, have children—and have a husband who would single-handedly
provide for them. Many saw work as an interim step between school and
marriage/children. It would seem that the women's movement has yet to have
a dramatic impact on young working class girls. On the contrary I sensed

a type of backlash from girls with working mothers. They planned to be home for their children so that they could provide the kinds of emotional and physical support (milk and cookies at 3:00 p.m.) that they felt was missing in their childhood. It might very well be that these girls are in a transitional stage in their lives, that they will be able to recognize the economical and emotional benefits that they were afforded through a working mother later in their adulthood. (Let us hope so!)

Other Obstacles

External or societal barriers soon become another set of variables that inhibit achievement and career motivation in women. They are not easily differentiated from those already mentioned; in fact, many women have internalized them to the extent that they no longer perceive them as external barriers at all—instead they search inside themselves to see what they are doing "wrong," how they are inciting others to act in a particular way, *ad nauseam*. Discrimination on the job and in hiring, co-worker and supervisor attitudes, salary inequities, suggested academic curriculum and sex-biased career testing, are just some of the factors that can become barriers to women's career development. However, I will not take the time here to explore these obstacles as they have been challenged many times elsewhere in the literature. I do want to stress that these forces remain with us and their effects, both subtle and overt, continue to take their toll on women today.

Some Implications

Thus far I have described some of the factors that may be influencing a woman's career decision-making process. In my own practice as a career counselor I have found that when I am working with women I could not assume, as most theorists would suggest, that their age or economic/social status would dictate where they were in their vocational process. Unlike men who have been found to have specific developmental stages according to age, women have their own developmental process. A majority are in a much earlier stage than has been normed for their age. Indeed, I would postulate that developmentally they are still in the fantasy or tentative choice stage that most theorists have ascribed to adolescents. Thus, although they are functioning as adults in many ways with its inherent responsibilities and rewards, vocationally they have a lot of discovering and thinking to do. They need the opportunity to go through the clarifying, exploring and choice-making steps that most theorists assume have taken place during their adolescence. But, unfortunately, for most women this does not happen. They are going to need help in gathering information about a wide range of career choices; they need to do the self-assessment which will help them to discover their interests, values, skills, needs. But even before they tackle any of these steps, women have another set of issues that needs to be recognized.

When considering a career decision, many women must first explore their internal issues of ambivalence and commitment, their fears of both success and failure, and their needs for affiliation as well as for power and control. Relationships, with spouse/mate or among friends and family, also contribute to her inability to see her vocational goals clearly. It is only after taking the time to examine her present self-image and the significant influences on it that a woman will be able to build a positive self-concept so necessary to the career decision-making process.

Tools for Career Exploration

Most women facing career decisions assume that they are the only ones incapable of making a good clear decision. They experience a multitude of thoughts, feelings, anxieties and frustrations concerning their plight but they often feel burdensome to their friends and relatives if they talk to them. (Very often they choose not to even try since they feel that others cannot truly understand their situation.) Some women feel at a loss, stuck without any ideas or insights into the options available to them. And finally, some women are questioning their career commitment in general; for many the myth of Prince Charming is not dead—they secretly nurture fantasies of being taken care of when the right man comes along. I have found that working together in a group is a powerful and effective means of exploring these and other issues that can hold women back from making progress in their vocational development.

Successful groups challenge that subtle but pervasive myth that we are all individuals who must conquer the world alone, even it if means stepping on some fingers and toes along the way. Becoming a part of a group, being stimulated, pushed, motivated, and excited, becomes an exhilarating learning experience. Co-members become teachers, role models, and authentic success stories. Motivation, direction and excitement actualize, empowering women's lives. They learn that they do not have to do it alone—there is a powerful force in working together as women.

I suggest that these groups take on a structure flexible in its ability to meet individual needs, while making sure it covers the basics of career decision-making. Although space does not permit a detailed guide to all that can be helpful and relevant to a women's support group I will briefly discuss what I have found to be the basics.

First, group dynamics need to be addressed. This includes member's needs and expectations so that members can be realistic about the goals of the group. Structure and commitment is discussed, including length and frequency of the meetings. A leader skilled in developing and facilitating groups can be useful in catalyzing group interaction; rotating leadership is another possibility.

Groups commonly run from 10–15 weeks, and I have facilitated groups which met for 6 months. I have found a division of five categories to be most helpful. The first few meetings come under the category of self-awareness; I call it Freeing Up Your Thinking. All too often women are so depressed by their job search that they have limited themselves before they have even begun. In my groups we do fantasy work, re-discover past accomplishments, and visualize the future.

The next section deals with three basic determinants of vocational choice—values, needs and interests. The goal here is to put vocational choice in perspective as a part of the woman's whole life instead of a separate piece.

Although skills assessment is most commonly lumped together with the previous section I have found it to be a very scary issue for many women and thus deserving of special attention. When considering their skills, most women will commonly negate or undervalue them. For some women this is a long and painful process; others will recognize and accept it as a challenge.

Now that women have become more aware of themselves they need to recognize the barriers and techniques to confront them. Risk-taking, decision-making, assertiveness training and secrets from the male locker room are all presented. This section engenders lively discussion and spontaneous brainstorming, as well as anger and frustration.

The final section puts mental discovery into action. Women discover first hand the advantages of the buddy system for keeping their motivation and spirits up. They set goals, explore alternatives, evaluate consequences. Verbal commitment becomes action.

FOOTNOTES

Lenore W. Harmon, "Career Counselling for Women," *Career Development and Counselling of Women*, eds. L. Sunny Hansen and Rita S. Rapoza, (Springfield, Ill: Charles Thomas, 1978), pg. 445.

Leona E. Tyler and Norman Sudberg, "Factors Affecting Career Choices of Adolescents" (University of Oregon: 1964) pg. 107-8.

Nancy Chodorow, "Being and Doing: A Cross Cultural Examination of the Socialization of Males and Females," *Women in Sexist Society*, eds. Vivian Gornick and Barbara Moran, (Basic Books, N.Y., 1971), pg. 272.

Kay F. Schaffer, *Sex Roles and Human Behavior*, (Cambridge, Mass.; Winthrop Publishers, 1981). pg. 155.

REFERENCES

Bloom, Lynn A., Karen Coburn, and Joan Pearlman. *The New Assertive Woman*, New York: Dell Publishing Co., 1975.

Burtle, Vasantie and Violet Franks. *Women in Therapy*, New York: Brunner/Mazel, 1974.

Fleming, Patricia J. *Beyond Coping: How to Form a Vocational Support Group for Women*, Boston, 1979.

Hansen, L. Sunny and Rita S. Rapoza. *Career Development and Counselling of Women*. Springfield, Illinois: Charles C Thomas, 1979.

Hennig, Margaret and Ann Jardim. *The Managerial Women*, New York: Anchor Press/Doubleday, 1976.

Holland, John. *Making Vocational Choices: A Theory of Careers*, New Jersey: Prentice-Hall, 1973.

Mednick, M. T. S., S. S. Tangri, and Hoffman. *W. D. C. Hemisphere*, "Women and Achievements; Social and Motivational Analysis." 1975.

Miller, Jean Baker. *Towards a New Psychology of Women*, Boston; Beacon Press, 1976.

Nemerowicz, Gloria Morris. *Children's Perceptions of Gender and Work Roles*, New York: Praeger Publishers, 1979.

Osipow, Samuel H. *Theories of Career Development*, New Jersey; Prentice-Hall, 1973.

Roe, Anne. *Psychology of Occupations*, New York: John Wiley and Sons, Inc., 1956.

Scarf, Maggie. *Unfinished Business: Pressure Points in the Lives of Women*, New York: Doubleday, 1980.

Schaffer, Kay F. *Sex Roles and Human Behavior*, Cambridge, Mass.: Winthrop Publishers, 1981.

Scholz, Nelle Tumlin, Judith Sissbee Prince and Gordon Porter Miller. *How to Decide: A Workbook for Women*, New York: Avon, 1975.

Super, Donald. *The Psychology of Careers*, New York: Harper and Row, 1957.

Tyler, Leona E. and Norman Subberg. *Factors Affecting Career Choices of Adolescents*, University of Oregon, 1964.

TRANSFORMING BODY IMAGE:
YOUR BODY, FRIEND OR FOE?

Marcia Germaine Hutchinson

It is a sad truth, but the great majority of women in our culture do not accept their bodies. There is hardly a woman in this country who has not at some time in her life chastised and tortured herself for being too fat, too thin, not pretty enough, too flat-chested, too buxom, too hairy, too old, too flabby, etc., etc.. The list could and does go on. It is a rare woman who lives in a state of peace and harmony with her body.

In this article I will share some of the findings of a research project in which I studied the phenomenon of negative body image in thirty physically and psychologically healthy women of normal weight between the ages of 24 and 40 years. This report will include a discussion of this psycho-cultural issue as well as a summary of a treatment intervention which I created and tested on a sample of these women all of whom presented themselves as disliking or denying their bodies. For a more complete presentation I refer the reader to my original study (Sankowsky, 1981).

Body image is a very subtle and complex phenomenon referring to the organized subjective experience and mental representation of the body. It encompasses sensations, proprioceptive awareness, feelings, and attitudes toward the body. Body-cathexis is the value-laden aspect of the body image experience that describes the degree of satisfaction or dissatisfaction with the body. Body image is not the same as the body, but is rather what the mind does to the body in translating the experience of embodiment into its mental representation. This translation from body to body image and from there to body-cathexis is a complex and emotionally charged process.

When the body image is negative it can manifest on a continuum from complete dissociation or denial of the body to open warfare with the whole or parts of the body. The body has become the symbol or target for everything that is wrong in life and the object of intense judgment, contempt, and shame.

What appears to be at the heart of negative body image is a state of disem-

Marcia Germaine Hutchinson is a body-centered psychotherapist in the Boston area. She has an individual and group practice working with body image issues and teaches in the Counseling Psychology Department at Leslie College, Cambridge, MA.

bodiment. The body is experienced as alien and lost to awareness or as an adversary—two sides of the coin of disembodiment. Somewhere there has occurred a loss of the sense of integrity. The body has broken away or has been severed from the mind and is experienced as a foreign object, an albatross, or a hated antagonist. It becomes something to ignore, deny, deprive or otherwise whip into shape or get under control. The pain of separation of mind and body ranges from the dull ache of deadness and depression to the excruciation of self-torture.

Negative body image is reaching epidemic proportions in the American female population. It seriously intrudes into the sphere of life significantly affecting same and opposite sex relationships, the capacity for intimacy and sexual expression, psychological and physical health and self-caring practices, professional development, personal expression, projection, and fulfillment. It impacts psychological functioning with consuming feelings of self-doubt, fear, worry, self-contempt, depression, shame, guilt, and lowered self-esteem. And yet, this is a clinical issue which has to date received little attention from the male-dominated psychological community, their preference being to ignore it, or dismiss it as superficial and a symptom of deeper psychopathology. What is missing is an examination of the cultural context in which this "symptom" flourishes.

We live in a culture that places a high value on beauty, appearance, and outer image. If this is true for our culture as a whole, it is doubly true for its women. Although the Women's Movement has succeeded to some degree in changing and expanding the role possibilities for women, the truth remains that the majority of women alive today are the products of less enlightened socialization styles. These strategies, so deeply embedded in the fabric of the American culture, would have us believe that woman's chief, and perhaps only, role is as ornament, wife, and mother. Fundamental to carrying out her expected role and its consequent fulfillment is the condition that she be attractive enough to snare a mate who can give her the opportunity to live out her biological and social destiny. Thus to be fulfilled in life a woman learns that she must have at least a modicum of that highly prized commodity known as physical beauty.

It is the adequacy and attractiveness of her body that seals a woman's fate, that assures her future acceptance and security, that dictates to a certain degree her level of satisfaction or dissatisfaction with the course of her life. Or so the myth goes. It is this body-self-role parallel—the identification of a woman with her body—that sets the stage for this enormous charge that so many women carry around their bodies and their attractiveness as well as for the impact that body image distortion has on self-image.

When I set out to study this issue I sought subjects with no history of psychiatric illness or eating disorder. It immediately became clear that it is a rare woman in this culture who is not eating disordered or who does not experience herself as struggling with food and weight issues. Of 114 women screened for this study 109 reported an unnatural relationship to food and eating. Of those selected as subjects—whose weights all fell within the normal range—only one woman was not actively waging a war against fat. This astonishing statistic suggests that weight and eating issues are inseparable from body image struggles in today's woman.

Although describing themselves as eating disordered, when queried further most women reported eating patterns typical of the culture as a whole, patterns that in men would never be labelled as pathological. These women are for the most part suffering not from eating disorders but from labelling disorders.

We live in a culture where fat has become Public Enemy Number One and dieting a national obsession. The last 25 to 30 years have been witness to three parallel cultural developments that have helped to make eating disorders and negative body image household words: the weight-watching/fitness movement; the rise of the media; and the Women's Movement.

In 1959 a major medical study linking longevity and health with thinness resulted in a major readjustment of the height-weight tables. Normal weight people woke up to discover that they had become 10–15 pounds overweight overnight! A giant weight and fitness industry was born and with it a national mania for thinness. Any amount of "extra" poundage carried on the body's frame has come to be seen as the outward manifestation of deep character flaws, lack of self-caring, and slow suicide. The same dynamic that is feeding the frightening rise of anorexia and bulimarexia—diseases characterized by distortions of the body image and disordered eating behavior—in the female population is in a milder but more pervasive way at work in those women who struggle with the acceptability of their bodies. Recent medical studies of equal rigor strongly suggest that longevity and health correlate with extra poundage rather than extra leanness. The height-weight tables have been returned to their pre-1959 level. It remains to be seen whether our cultural insanity can be reversed. This very complex subject of weight and eating can be studied further in the works of Chernin (1981), Millman (1980), Orbach (1978), and Bruch (1973).

Another powerful cultural force in this picture is the media. Although films and fashion magazines have been influencing the cultural norm that defines feminine beauty for many years, it is only since the advent and mass availability of television that the media has become such an unprecedentedly powerful agent of cultural transmission. Not a single woman that I have interviewed about this subject (approximately 125) has failed to acknowledge the role of the media in transmitting and propagating cultural standards of beauty. Today's woman is constantly reminded—by a dizzying succession of media images and their impact on the public taste—of how she measures up or fails to measure up to the unreal, restrictive, elusive and ephemeral aesthetic standard of the time.

Raised to be other-directed, women have tended to operate from an external frame of reference looking to the outside for cues about who they are, how to be, how to look, whether they are adequate or inadequate, and about how to think of themselves. The comparison of self and body to cultural images as well as to family and peers is the context in which a woman defines herself and her worth. Media images are in themselves powerful and women have been especially receptive and vulnerable to them.

The media plays a powerful role in yet another tyranny. Americans, especially women, are continually bombarded by opposing and equally powerful messages from the media—television, radio, periodicals, and advertising—which on the one hand extol the virtues of thinness and decry the obscenity of fat, while on the other hand stimulate the digestive juices with appetizing morsels to eat. This is a classical case of the double-bind. Caught between the requirement to be thin, fit, and beautiful and a world full of eating opportunities is it any wonder that eating has become an "issue" rather than a simple, life-supporting pleasure?

Today's women, having been told by the medical profession that her normal weight—the weight that her body naturally gravitates toward—is too much, feels guilty, ashamed, and out of control. She then either eats more to dull the pain or tries to diet, starve, or otherwise whip her body into the desired size and shape. But the stress is too great and the regime too rigorous. The body will not be so easily denied and a pattern of compulsive overeating takes the place of stringent dieting and the feelings of guilt and shame return. And so the cycle goes.

Into this already complex cultural scenario we must add one further conflicting voice—that of the Women's Movement. This voice tells women not to minimize themselves, but rather to be more, to be larger, to be powerful. Caught between these contradictory messages and pressure—eat/don't eat; be more/be less—it should come as no surprise that a woman's body has become a battlefield on which this war is being fought.

What determines whether a woman's body becomes her home or a warzone? We all grow up under similar cultural influences, and yet not all women dislike or disown their bodies. Having studied this issue only in a sample of women who struggle with it, I cannot draw solid conclusions about the developmental features that differentiate this group from women who have neutral or positive attitudes about their bodies. Some common developmental themes emerged from my study.

In some cases the distortion of the body image came early in life with inadequate touching or poor handling of the body by significant objects. These women had no memories of ever feeling at home in their bodies. Their bodies had never been affirmed by the loving, caring touch of parental figures.

The body images of significant family role model—especially mother and father—play a powerful role in shaping a child's body image. Parental valuation or devaluation of their own bodies—usually communicated non-verbally through body language—is an important factor in the child's learning to accept or reject her own body and its functions. It is common for a woman to incorporate a family body image—and especially her mother's body image into her own, for better or for worse.

An abundance of criticism and a dearth of positive reinforcement beginning early in life set the stage for later self-criticism and feelings of bodily inadequacy. Nagging and ridiculing parental comments about weight, eating behavior, and clothing were often internalized, echoing for years to come. Many women noted an overinvolvement by the mother in the affairs of their body creating a strong emotional charge and weakening the sense of ownership of their own bodies.

Although the age of onset for negative body image was variable, most of the women in this study noted puberty as the turning point in their relationship with their bodies. At best puberty is a time of bodily awkwardness, rapid change, and body image confusion. It is at this time that we feel exquisitely whether we and our bodies fit in or fail to do so. The experiences and messages surrounding the body for many women become stuck or "frozen" into the body image at this time when our bodies are developing and transforming us from little girls to nubile young women. This process for most of the women in this study was fraught with awkwardness, feelings of inadequacy and fears of sexuality, power, and individuation. For many this burgeoning womanliness was something to be hidden either by burying it under layers of fat, or by excessive dieting to deny the existence of any womanly curves.

For some puberty meant the beginning of competition with the mother. For most it marked a significant shift in the father-daughter relationship. Some fathers gave tacit messages through their own discomfort that it was not safe or acceptable to be pretty and sexual, that it would lead to rejection and withdrawal or sexual invasion.

Puberty marked the time of entry into the sexual "marketplace" where scarcity of supply demanded excellence and spelled pressure and competition with peers. Lessons learned here about attractiveness, desirability, and "salability" were lessons difficult to unlearn.

So it can be seen that body image development is a complex and variable phenomenon in which the family—the mouthpiece for cultural values—plants the seeds of negativity which the culture later cultivates.

It was the major purpose of my study to create and test the effectiveness of a treatment intervention designed to help women become more accepting and compassionate toward their bodies. The results of the experiment were dramatically positive, both quantitative and qualitative measures indicating significant improvement in both body and self image. Subsequent work with additional women has supported the power of the treatment in transforming a woman's relationship to her body.

The therapy consists of eight weekly group meetings involving a focused application of active Guided Imagery or Visualization used in conjunction with a journal process. The assumption that body image is itself an image suggested the use of controlled imaging as the appropriate tool for accessing and altering the subjective experience of the body. The journal process provided a means for each woman to process her imagined experience, translating it from right cerebral hemisphere (image) to left (language).

The work consisted to each woman's deep, personal, private exploration and processing of her own material. As group leader I functioned in the role of imagery guide providing the instruction for inner travel. The group provided support through shared focus and energy. Group processing was minimal so that each participant would be directed inward to contact her own power and her own answers.

Imagery as a clinical tool is currently enjoying a renaissance. Since image is the language of the unconscious, the focused use of imagery is capable of arousing deep affect with economy and gentleness. It accesses those recesses of the psyche where primary-process and affective memories are stored. Its subtle, non-intrusive, and often symbolic character circumvents defensiveness and resistance. Focused imaging can create new mental patterns and attitudes. Through the manipulation of images an individual can gain access to and control of cognitive maps—such as the body image—that manifest in destructive attitudes, moods, and compulsive behavior patterns.

In general, the treatment takes the following stance: The work is not about changing your body, but about learning to love the body you have. The emphasis is on helping each woman own her uniqueness of body and self and to choose to be kinder and more accepting of herself.

The broad objectives of the treatment intervention were as follows:

1. To use imagery as a means of accessing and reworking buried historical and emotional material relating to body image development.
2. To convey a sense of the power of the imagination in shaping reality as well as a sense of each woman's power in manipulating and controlling her own imagery including body imagery.
3. To heighten awareness of the blockages to change—resistance, fear, attachment to old images, defenses and attitudes—and to provide methods for transcending these barriers.
4. To enhance a sense of embodiment by maintaining an intense and tenacious focus on the body, its history, its movement patterns, and body language as well as to forge a deeper and more compassionate communication between mind and body.
5. To bring about an attitudinal shift toward the body by clearing a space for new positive, healing imagery creating a new experience of respect and positive regard for the body.

The design of the workshop is progressive, each step building on the learning and clearing accomplished in the previous step. Following is a brief outline of the eight sessions:

Session 1. Training the imagination.

Session 2. Developing kinesthetic awareness, a detailed mapping of the body image including area of emotional charge. Willful distortion and manipulation of the body image in order to impart a sense of control over the subjective experience of the body.

Session 3. Exploring family roots including family body images, the impact of parents and significant role models on the valuation of the body. Rewriting key psycho-historical events using adult resources and imaginal confrontation with important figures from the past.

Session 4. Exploring critical introjects incorporated in the body image. Dialoguing with disowned or negatively-cathected body parts.

Session 5. Disidentification process examining the nature of the attachment to negative body imagery and experimenting with letting go of these identifications. Experimentation with new body images, postures, movement patterns, and attitudes.

Session 6. An imagined escape from the body image as symbolic prison. An imaginal massage where, through the healing of her own touch, energy is transferred from positively- to negatively-cathected body areas. Real and imaginal mirror affirmation work.

Session 7. Negotiation with the Saboteur, the voice of resistance and sabotage. Creation of a metaphor representing the process of the gradual adoption of a new body image.

Session 8. Processing, sharing, and closing.

Guided Imagery is a subtle, profound, and respectful way of working with the psyche. The judicious and clinically well-grounded uses of mental imagery can provide a powerful key for unlocking the doors to the unconscious where important material lies waiting to be exposed to the light of awareness. This therapeutic approach also offers a non-threatening, gentle approach to creating new psychological maps that can serve the individual in establishing a more fulfilling style of living.

Not only did the majority of women in this study experience significant changes in their feelings about themselves and their bodies, but they also rediscovered and honed the imaginal faculty through disciplined use. The imagination was discovered by them to be a powerful resource and ally in heightening awareness, exploring the past, changing history, and creating new cognitive maps and psychic attitudes.

Negative body image is a clinical issue of considerable magnitude that is only now beginning to receive the attention it deserves. Most people in this culture are subject to the cultural values surrounding the body. For the female half of the population these values are intimately married to her sense of self. Whether the body becomes the target of an unacceptable self or the reverse is a dilemma of the chicken-egg variety. But it becomes a moot question when the intimate body-self connection for women is kept in mind.

It is essential that clinicians who treat women clients be cognizant of the importance of a positive body image in female well-being. It is the responsibility of these clinicians to be willing and knowledgeable enough to guide their clients in unravelling the mysteries that surround the relationship with the body and to foster the separation from old, internalized destructive patterns and the adoptions of new, life-serving programs of bodily and self-esteem.

Negative body image in women is a phenomenon that has its roots simultaneously in many soils. It is a physical phenomenon created out of bodily experiences and in turn impacting the well-being of the physical organism itself. It is a psychological phenomenon woven out of the threads of personal history, expressed as a distortion of the imagination, and changeable through the agency of that same part of the psyche. It is a cultural phenomenon in a culture that perpetuates the myth that there is one way for a woman to look, and that socializes into its female members a drive to conform to these standards. It is a political phenomenon embodying a form of political oppression whereby women waste enormous amounts of energy and human potential locked in a struggle with their bodies, potential that could better be used in developing other aspects of their beings. Lastly, it is a philosophical-spiritual phenomenon endorsed and reinforced by much religious training and the Cartesian duality that splits the self off from the body creating of it a target, a symbol of the enemy.

REFERENCES

Bruch, H. Eating disorders. New York: Basic Books, 1973.
Chernin, K. The obsession: reflections on the tyranny of slenderness. New York: Harper & Row, 1981.
Millman, M. Such a pretty face. New York: W. W. Norton, 1980.
Orbach, S. Fat is a feminist issue. New York: Paddington Press, 1978.
Sankowsky, M. The effect of a treatment based on the use of guided visuo-kinesthetic imagery on the alteration of negative body-cathexis in women. Unpublished doctoral dissertation, Boston University, 1981.

BATTERED WOMEN, CULTURAL MYTHS AND CLINICAL INTERVENTIONS: A FEMINIST ANALYSIS

Michele Bograd

Sexist biases in conventional clinical theory and in our culture at large shape clinical interventions with battered women. Many battered women seek treatment in traditional mental health settings even though clinical theory and technique are of limited applicability to the distinct concerns of these women. The significant and substantial feminist writings on the politics of woman abuse have been almost disregarded in the current development of clinical literature on battered women. Analysis from a feminist perspective reveals that clinical approaches to battered women are based less on scientific formulation and research than on prevailing male-defined cultural myths about women. By integrating feminist views with a balanced clinical perspective, this article will demonstrate some of the ways cultural myths influence clinical interventions with battered women. Because these myths are so ingrained in the world view of male and female therapists, the evaluation of personal assumptions is a prerequisite to treating battered women. For this reason, this article focuses on how therapists think about battering and women, rather than on treatment strategies or models. Common clinical misconceptions will be challenged and useful reconceptualization of major issues in the identification/diagnosis and treatment of battered women will be presented.

Identification and Diagnosis of Battered Women

Myths are unquestioned beliefs embodying popular ideas concerning natural or historical phenomena that function to validate and support the existing social order (Oakley, 1974). Myths which perpetuate woman abuse

Ms. Bograd is a doctoral candidate, University of Chicago. She is currently in private practice in Cambridge, MA and provides consultation and training on woman abuse. The author wishes to thank the staff members of the Family Service Unit in Quincy, MA, particularly Ms. Leah Freed, for their support and critical comments of earlier drafts of this article.

Address reprint requests to Ms. Bograd, Riverside Psychological Associates, 334 Broadway, Cambridge, MA 02139.

include: 1. battering is a rare phenomenon; 2. women are battered because of their presumed psychopathology; 3. women are responsible for their victimization by male partners; 4. violence is an expectable if not acceptable part of female experience. These myths exert a powerful influence on the early identification and diagnosis of battered women.

Few women, even those who have suffered physical abuse, identify themselves as battered women (Bograd, note l). Most agencies omit standardized intake questions concerning abuse and clinicians don't systematically probe for its occurrence. This is due in part to the myths that battering is a deviant and uncommon act and that violence within limits is an integral part of women's relationships. In fact, it is part of *many* women's lives: a national study revealed that one out of four women will experience an incident of abuse over the course of her marriage (Straus, Gelles & Steinmetz, 1980). Cultural myths often deter clinicians from probing for abuse or lead them to pose value-laden questions (i.e., what did you do to make him so angry?) Because of this, battered women are not identified as such in clinical interviews. When battering *is* identified during initial interviews, careful diagnosis can be compromised or misdirected by unthinking allegiance to myths about battered women. This occurs in two ways: 1. by minimizing the violence; 2. by misusing clinical constructs to account for it.

Clinicians often minimize information that a woman has been slapped on occasion because they subscribe to the widespread myth that some physical harm, particularly if it is "mild" and "infrequent," is a "natural" or "normal" part of marriage (Gelles, 1972; Straus, 1980). This denies the terror and intimidation battered women must cope with even in periods of relative marital calm. Battering can also be minimized by defining it simply as part of the social context. Battered women often present a number of psychosocial problems including alcoholic husbands, behavioral problems with their children, traumatic childhood histories and multiple losses (Gayford, 1975a, 1975b; Martin, 1976; Rounsaville, 1978; Scott, 1974). As clinicians construct narratives of the woman's life, abuse can be integrated as "one problem among many" or as a "logical" outcome of life stresses. The abuse is hidden and redefined as something else: its presence virtually disappears as a real and determining factor in the woman's life (Stark & Flicraft, note 2). A strong feminist position suggests that the woman's terror and brutalization are *primary* clinical problems and must be addressed as such.

The misuse of clinical constructs to account for battering also derives from cultural myths. In diagnostic formulations, battering is often defined as a secondary problem or as evidence of a woman's "more basic" psychological dysfunction: she is beaten because she is depressed, paranoid or borderline (Gillman, 1980). Effect is confounded with cause: she may be depressed or paranoid because she is abused. There is no empirical evidence to date documenting whether her symptoms may dissipate once she is free from danger (Walker, 1980). But the social learning theory of learned helplessness (Walker, 1977-78, 1979) and the psychodynamic theories of traumatic psychological infantilism (A. Symonds, 1975) and the stress response syndrome (Hilberman, 1980; Hilberman & Munson, 1977-78) suggest the battered woman's symptoms are directly attributable to her abuse. Conclusive diagnoses of psychopathology can be made only after violence has been addressed in treatment. Some battered women may exhibit underlying psychopathology. This shouldn't influence clinical judgment of the abuse as a real problem, however, unless one agrees with the myth that a woman is beaten because she's crazy.

A more insidious misuse of clinical constructs links abuse directly to the woman's personality through the motivational construct of masochism: battering gratifies psychological needs based on intrapsychic conflicts engendered in the distant past (Reynolds & Siegle, 1959; Shainess, 1977, 1979; Snell, Rosenwalk & Robey, 1964). Enlightened clinicians have replaced this formulation with the equally damaging notion of provocation: the woman asks for it. Careful analysis reveals that "provocation" is a male-defined term used by male partners to describe any of the woman's behaviors that precede the abuse which the men judge as overstepping the boundaries of the proper wife (Dobash & Dobash, 1979) "Masochism" refers to individual psychological needs as sufficient explanation for battering while ignoring the immobilizing external social constraints that trap battered women in abusive relationships (Gelles, 1976; Waites, 1977-78). Used indiscriminately, these clinical constructs are meaningless when applied to the battered woman.

Though clinical formulations have an important place in interventions with battered women, even well-intentioned formulations compound their victimization. Diagnoses of characterological dsyfunction prevent clinicians from recognizing that some women remain in abusive relationships because they view their marriages as more desirable than their limited alternatives (Goodstein & Page, 1981; Pfouts, 1978). The woman's adaptive responses to her situation can be misinterpreted as dysfunctional symptoms stemming from intra-psychic factors rather than as survival mechanisms. This leads clinicians to focus on the hidden psychological meanings of the violence (i.e., why does the woman need to be punished?) rather than on the abuse as violation of her physical integrity.

Clinical theory reflects the myth that "provocation" is adequate justification for violence, that violence is permissible if the woman is at fault. And where is the abusive male in clinical theory and formulation? Little clinical literature exists on the abusive male which in itself reflects the male bias in research on battering. Though there is evidence to suggest that some men exhibit psychopathology (Faulk, 1974, 1977; M. Symonds, 1978), the proportion of men who batter family members and suffer from psychological disorders is no greater than the proportion of the population-at-large with psychological disorders (Straus, 1980). By defining public social concerns as private psychiatric problems, the diagnostic labeling of either partner reinforces the erroneous myth that battering is uncommon and limited to a disturbed or deviant population. A feminist perspective states that woman abuse is due less to the psychopathology of either partner and more to the unequal power relations between men and women in our society which accepts violence as the ultimate and legitimate resource of husbands (McCormack, 1980).

Myths and Treatment Strategies

Traditional clinical training and theory are of limited relevance for intervention in cases with overt violence against women because, until recently, woman abuse wasn't addressed as a serious dilemma for the field. While critical comment on various treatment strategies is beyond the scope of this paper, this section will suggest how unquestioned acceptance of myths about battered women leads to inappropriate treatment strategies particularly: 1. ignoring violence as a primary treatment issue; 2. the incorrect allocation of responsibility for the violence.

Violence as a primary treatment issue. It is easy to ignore violence as a primary treatment issue as diagnostic formulations and cultural myths deflect attention onto the battered woman and away from her situation, her partner and the violence itself. Abusive men and battered women also tend to minimize the extent or severity of the violence while clinicians feel more comfortable and competent treating other issues—be they depression or anxiety in the individual or poor communication patterns and structure in the couple. Lack of direct intervention with the violence is equivalent to an implicit acceptance of violence as either normative or understandable in marriage. The failure to recognize that the battered woman is in crisis because of the violence may result in coercive and inappropriate treatment. For example, medication and hospitalization may numb and further isolate the woman so reducing her coping skills before her return to a partner who continues to be violent (Walker, 1979). Treatment strategies based on the assumption that violence results from dysfunctional individual or couples patterns are equally ineffective in controlling the violence. After months in treatment, a couple may learn to communicate well even as the man may remain episodically violent. Furthermore, unless the violence is addressed, the successful treatment of other clinical issues will also be limited. For example, in order to bring a distant and abusive husband into closer contact with his wife, a clinician prescribed tasks to increase their intimacy without taking into account how impossible it was for the wife to trust her unpredictable violent husband (Bograd, note 3). Clinical interventions around any individual or couples problems are frequently ineffective until the violence is directly confronted by the therapist.

As violence organizes the life of the couple, so will it organize treatment. While some authors have stated that the "aggressive" aspects of the relationship may be treated concurrently with other issues (Goodstein & Page, 1981), this presupposes that a viable treatment alliance has been established. But a clinician cannot be assured of the alliance while the man is actively violent with his partner. Abusive men typically agree to treatment for reasons other than to control their violence. They may be motivated by a desire to reconcile with their wives or to monitor what information is discussed during sessions. A treatment alliance can't be established with a man who isn't committed to dealing with his violence and who seeks to control the therapy (Walker, 1981). The battered woman will be guarded in treatment, in spite of ostensible cooperation, because she knows the therapist can't protect her (Walker, 1981). Until she is safe to work in treatment without fear of retaliation from her partner, the therapeutic alliance will be further compromised. For these reasons, the violence must be named and dealt with as the primary treatment issue. This requires that clinicians evaluate how their implicit assumptions about violence against women influence their treatment strategies.

Incorrect allocation of responsibility for the violence. Concerning treatment strategies, practical considerations frequently shape recommendations of individual treatment for the battered woman. She is symptomatic and appears for treatment while her abusive partner experiences little psychological distress and rarely seeks treatment until the woman threatens to leave him. Reference to such practical impediments often conceal the myths that women are battered because of their presumed psychopathology and are responsible for their partners' violent behaviors. These myths reflect cultural definitions of women as caretakers of men's emotions and as solely accountable for the tranquility of the domestic environment. Individual treatment is prescribed for the battered woman because she is defined as the locus of the problem. While a battered woman may find some relief in long-term individual psychotherapy, such a strategy has no impact on controlling her partner's abusive behavior. Labelling her the identified patient may foster a maladaptive dependency on the therapist (Ridington, 1977–78; Ball & Wyman, 1977–78). It also compounds the battered woman's guilt and low self-esteem while reinforcing her erroneous belief that she is responsible for the abuse. Battered women in treatment are particularly vulnerable to such labelling because women who have internalized prevalent myths and so blame themselves for their partners' violent behaviors are twice as likely to seek psychotherapy as women who blame their partners (Frieze, 1979).

While individual treatment is often prescribed for battered women, many clinicians prefer interventions based on family systems theories such as marital therapy. While systems formulations may illuminate patterns in violent relationships (Hanks & Rosenbaum, 1977; Margolin, 1979; Saunders, 1977), this doesn't mean that couples treatment is the strategy of choice (Fleming, 1979; Star, Clark, Goetz, & O'Malia, 1979; Walker, 1979). While couples treatment appears to shift responsibility for the abuse to the male, it commonly reinforces myths about women's responsibility for the abuse. Systems theories share an emphasis on functional explanations of human behavior: all interdependent parts serve a role in maintaining the homeostatic balance of a system. Functional explanations of battering, however, are often confused with moral judgments. The formulation that partners interact in specific patterned ways to maintain a violent marital system is *not* equivalent to the statement that each is equally responsible for the violence. Though one can caution that it is not "pejorative" to recognize that a woman (allegedly) plays a major role in her abuse (Lion, 1977), the fine line between supposedly neutral clinical recognition of systemic patterns and judgmental allocation of blame is often impossible to discern.

Family systems theories interact with cultural definitions of male and female nature. Anger is a legitimate if not valued emotion for men in our society who are viewed as having emotional thresholds beyond which they exert no control. Because male violence is commonly viewed as reactive, rather than as proactive behavior to gain dominance or control, the focus in couples treatment becomes the woman's behaviors. Myths about the role of men and women during violent incidents further implicate the woman. In a recent exploratory study, Washburn, Frieze and Knoble (note 4) found that mental health professionals believed that the majority of battered women intentionally or unconsciously provoke the violence while they viewed the majority of men prone to beat women as doing it unintentionally. Ironically, when abusive men account for their use of physical force with their partners, they contradict these cultural myths: While denying their actions were violent, they often report they *did* intend to hurt their partners (Bograd, note 1). Treatment strategy, clinical theory and cultural myths interact to support the male's tendency to deny his primary role in violent marital incidents.

Therapists further collude with this denial if they believe they cannot categorically tell a woman she doesn't contribute to the violence. Goodstein & Page (1981) state this prevents exploration of a woman's behaviors which may lead to her being abused in the future. While it is important to help the battered woman develop coping skills, there is a subtle but crucial difference between suggesting that the woman modify her behavior to protect herself given the inevitability of the violence and blaming her for contributing to if not initiating future violent incidents. Focusing on the woman's contribution again shifts responsibility onto her, reinforces her belief that she can and should accommodate her behavior to her partner's demands, and supports her illusion of control. The therapist must convey to the battered woman that she is ultimately powerless to prevent her partner's violence; that many women are battered; that she is not crazy; and that no woman deserves to be beaten. The myths about battered women need to be named and explicitly defined as untrue.

Feminist Theory and Clinical Work with Battered Women

Cultural myths interact with clinical theory to conserve traditional images of women even as they conceal the gender- and role-specific character of violence against wives. This article has presented a feminist analysis of some of the ways that socially created myths about women battering influence clinical interventions ranging from intake procedures to treatment strategies. The uncritical acceptance of these myths blocks clinical understanding of the causes and dynamics of battering, rationalizes conventional interventions, and functions to maintain the violence and the privileged position of the male partner.

As therapists become sensitive to how their work with battered women is shaped by cultural myths, they often experience an unnerving jolt of recognition, a sense of disorientation as they question their theoretical models and everyday assumptions about male/female relations, and feelings of despair as they acknowledge the massive social changes necessary to end violence against women. But a feminist critique need not imply that all clinical work with battered women is misguided or without value.

Among other things, feminist analysis reveals the relationship between cultural myths, clinical theory and the personal problems of individual women. A feminist analysis describes the social and historical dimensions of the subordination of women and demonstrates how the beliefs which codify male dominance also promote violence against women. But feminist theory is not clinical theory. Some radical feminists argue that psychotherapy is an inappropriate or coercive intervention for battered women. But as long as battered women continue to turn to mental health agencies, it is essential that feminists continue to identify the myths influencing clinical theory and practice. Feminist clinicians can provide analyses of the complex interaction of individual psyche and social situations, develop sensitive and politically enlightened models of intervention, and alleviate the distress of many battered women. Though the application and extension of feminist analyses to current clinical practice with battered women, psychotherapy can serve as a valuable intermediate tool of change even as other feminists work to transform the social conditions of women's lives.

REFERENCE NOTES

1. Bograd, M. *Conjugal violence as rule-governed action: The understanding of abusive and non-abusive persons.* Doctoral dissertation in preparation, 1982.

2. Stark. E., & Flicraft, A. *Therapeutic intervention as a situational determinant of the battering syndrome.* Paper presented at the National Research Conference on Family Violence, Durham, New Hampshire, July, 1981.

3. Bograd, M. Personal communication during seminar with mental health professionals on clinical work with battered women, Quincy, MA, 1981.

4. Washburn, C., Frieze, I., & Knoble, J. *Some subtle biases of therapists towards women and violence.* Paper presented at the Annual Research Conference of the Association for Women in Psychology, Dallas, Texas, 1979.

REFERENCES

Ball, P., & Wyman, E. Battered wives and powerlessness: What can counselors do? *Victomology,* 2, 1977–78, 545–552.

Dobash, R. E., & Dobash, R. P. *Violence against wives: A case against the patriarchy.* New York: Free Press, 1979.

Faulk, M. Men who assault their wives. *Medicine, Science and the Law,* 1974, *14,*180–183.

Faulk, M. Men who assault their wives. In M. Roy (Ed.) *Battered women: A psychosocial study of domestic violence.* New York: Van Nostrand Reinhold Co., 1977.

Fleming, J. *Stopping wife abuse.* NY: Anchor Books, 1979.

Frieze, I. Perceptions of battered women. In I. Frieze, D. Bar-Tal & J. Carrol, *New approaches to social problems.* San Francisco: Jossey-Bass Publishers, 1979.

Gayford, J. Battered Wives.*Medicine, Science and the Law,* 1975, *15,* 237–245. (a)

Gayford, J. Wife battering: A preliminary study of 100 cases. *British Medical Journal,* 1975, *1,* 194–197. (b)

Gelles, R. *The violent home.* Beverly Hills, CA: Sage Publications, 1972.

Gelles, R. Abused wives: Why do they stay? *Journal of Marriage and the Family,* 1976, *38,* 659–668.

Gillman, J. An objective-relations approach to the phenomenon and treatment of battered women. *Psychiatry*, 1980, *43*, 346–358.

Goodstein, R., & Page, A. Battered wife syndrome: Overview of dynamics and treatment. *American Journal of Psychiatry*, 1981, *138*, 1036–1044.

Hanks, S., & Rosenbaum, C. Battered women: A study of women who live with violent and alcohol abusing men. *American Journal of Orthopsychiatry*, 1977, *47*, 291–306.

Hilberman, E. Overview: The "wife-beater's wife" reconsidered. *American Journal of Psychiatry*, 1980, *137*, 1336–1347.

Hilberman, E., & Munson, K. Sixty battered women. *Victimology*, 1977–78, *2*, 460–470.

Lion, J. Clinical aspects of wife-battering. In M. Roy (Ed.), *Battered women: A psychosocial study of domestic violence*. New York: Van Nostrand Reinhold Co., 1977.

Margolin, G. Conjoint marital therapy to enhance anger management and reduce spouse abuse. *American Journal of Family Therapy*, 1979, *7*, 13–24.

Martin, D. *Battered wives*. New York: Pocket Books, 1976.

McCormick, A. Men helping men stop woman abuse. *State and Mind*, Summer, 1980, 46–50.

Oakley, A. *Woman's work*. New York: Vintage Books, 1974.

Pfouts, J. Violent families: Coping responses of abused wives. *Child Welfare*, 1978, *57*, 101–111.

Reynolds, R., & Siegle, E. A study of casework with sado-masochistic marriage partners. *Social Casework*, 1959, *40*, 545–551.

Ridington, J. The transition process: A feminist environment as a reconstitutive milieu. *Victimology*, 1977–78, 563–575.

Rounsaville, B. Battered wives: Barriers to identification and treatment. *American Journal of Orthopsychiatry*, 1978, *48*, 487–494.

Saunders, D. Marital violence: Dimensions of the problem and modes of intervention. *Journal of Marriage and Family Counseling*, 1977, *12*, 43–52.

Scott, P. Battered wives. *British Journal of Psychiatry*, 1974, *125*, 433–441.

Shainess, N. Psychological aspects of wife battering. In M. Roy (Ed.), *Battered women: A psychosocial study of domestic violence*. New York: Van Nostrand Reinhold Co., 1977.

Shainess, N. Vulnerability to violence: Masochism as process. *American Journal of Psychotherapy*, 1979, *33*, 174–189.

Snell, J., Rosenwald, R., & Robey, A. The wifebeater's wife: A study of family interaction. *Archives of General Psychiatry*, 1964, *11*, 107–112.

Star, B., Clark, C., Goetz, K., & O'Malia, L. Psychosocial aspects of wife battering. *Social Casework*, 1979, *60*, 479–487.

Straus, M. A sociological perspective on the causes of family violence. In M. Geer (Ed.), *Violence and the Family*, Boulder, CO: Westview Press, 1980.

Straus, M. Victims and aggressors in marital violence. *American Behavioral Scientist*, 1980, *23*, 681–704.

Straus, M., Gelles, R., & Steinmetz, S. *Behind closed doors: Violence in the American family*. Garden City, N.Y.: Anchor Books, 1980.

Symonds, A. Violence against women—The myth of masochism. *American Journal of Psychotherapy*, 1979, *33*, 161–173.

Waites, E. Female masochism and the enforced restriction of choice. *Victimology*, 1977–78, *2*, 535–544.

Walker, L. Battered women and learned helplessness. *Victimology*, 1977–78, *2*, 525–534.

Walker, L. *The battered woman*. New York: Harper & Row, 1979.

Walker, L. Battered women. In A. Brodsky & R. Hare-Mustin (Eds.), *Women and psychotherapy*. New York: Guilford Press, 1980.

Walker, L. Battered women: Sex roles and clinical issues. *Professional Psychology*, 1981, *12*, 81–91.

SIBLING INCEST: THE MYTH OF BENIGN SIBLING INCEST

Ellen Cole

It is now established beyond all doubt that incest is prevalent in the United States. David Finklehor, author of *Sexually Victimized Children,* estimates that if the results of his survey of 796 college students were expanded to include non-college students, "about 40% of all women would have had some type of incestuous experience" (Good, 1981). The real taboo, until recently, has been not the act of incest, but the act of talking about it. An increasingly open discussion of incest is, however, resulting from a combination of updated reporting laws, and insistence from the feminist movement that crimes of violence against women be acknowledged.

The type of incest most widely discussed and researched, and most often reported to the authorities, is that between father and daughter (Herman, 1981). Generally believed to be the most commonly occurring type, however, is that between an older brother and a younger sister (Weeks, 1976; Finklehor, 1979). One author estimates that brother-sister incest is about five times more common than father-daughter incest in the general population (Lester, 1972). Yet little is written or known about sibling incest, probably because: 1. Reported cases are rare. Even if the victim tells, or the children are discovered, a parent is far less likely to "turn in" a son than a husband. Therefore, only 18% of arrests for incest are of brothers, compared to 78% of fathers (Francoeur, 1982). 2. It is believed that the consequences of sibling incest are often not damaging. Some writers think that sibling incest generally has little or no impact on either child (Strong et al., 1982; Lukianowicz, 1972); others agree that it can be harmful, but only if certain conditions are present, usually stated as an age difference of 5 years or more, or the use of physical force or coercion (Finklehor, 1979; Justice and Justice, 1978). The predominant belief, however, is that physical force is rare in sibling incest (Francoeur, 1982; Laredo, 1982). This article contends that sibling incest, when it involves an older brother and a younger sister, is not

---

Ellen Cole is a Vermont licensed practicing psychologist, and coordinator of psychological studies at Goddard College, in Plainfield, VT.

benign, even when the age difference is small and even when one or both of the participants report the experience as "positive."

It is important, of course, to distinguish between natural curiosity and exploration, on one hand, and harmful sibling incest, on the other. I agree with Forward and Buck (1978) when they say that "the game of show-me-yours-and-I'll-show-you-mine is older than civilization, and between young siblings of approximately the same age it is usually harmless." When the behaviors exceed the bounds of mutual and playful curiosity, however, the dynamics change. Neither the seriousness of sibling incest nor its complexity have been adequately appreciated, as can be understood from the following case descriptions.

Jenna

Jenna is a 20 year old, white college student. When she heard about my interest in sibling incest, she told me that she had been a victim, but it was too painful an experience for her to talk about. Instead, she gave me her journal to read, and we wrote several letters to each other. The following excerpts are presented here with her permission.

> I began to gain weight when I was 11 to keep my brother away. When I was 10 years old, and he was 15, he lured me into his bedroom for the first time by telling me that I could watch television with him, and that he wouldn't tell my parents. (I wasn't allowed to watch TV during the week). Part of me was intrigued when he asked me to take off my clothes. I touched my genitals every so often when I was younger. I didn't know what I was doing, but I knew it felt good, and I thought that taking my clothes off could hold some kind of pleasure. He had me sit in a chair, and I began to feel nervous when he tied me up tightly with the backs of my hands touching behind the chair, with rope tied around my wrists, my legs spread wide open, and my ankles tied to the legs of the chair. He took off his clothes and when I saw how large his penis was I was still somewhat intrigued but far too fearful. I asked him to untie me because the position I was in was uncomfortable and hurt, realizing to myself that my anticipation of pleasure had dissipated. I was scared. His response was simple and his voice was calm: "It would be no fair to me if I let you watch TV and don't tell, and I don't get to do anything without you telling." He has always

been the focus in the family. To this day he's babied by our parents. I feel closer to my brother than to anyone else in my family.

What's the difference between incest and rape? I feel I have been raped, and my life is ruined and tainted by it all the time. Not any part of me wants any person to see me as a woman. I have turned into a solid rock at the thought of an intimate relationship. I worked for four months at losing over 85 pounds, began to get involved in an intimate relationship, nearly had a nervous breakdown, and gained most of my weight back. I have turned down men who have genuinely cared about me by being brisk and bitchy at the first sign of intimacy. I know I have hurt them. In most cases after I was about 14 years old the sex I had was a selling of myself and nothing I could appreciate. Going through the motions.

Part of the reason I am so meticulously clean with my body and my belongings is because I feel dirty. I feel like dirt, smut. I always question if this incest is real. I talk myself into believing that it was just play between siblings. I force myself to be objective about it. I am afraid of how much anger and pain is there. I worry about people feeling sorry for me because I believe it was my fault and I don't deserve to be cared about. I've even convinced myself that the reason I hurt so much and the reason I'm so angry is because—how could I have done that to my brother?

Typical of incest of all types, Jenna and her brother did not have intercourse. Their sexual activities consisted mainly of manual and oral contact with the genitals, and less typically, of a high degree of sadistic and violent behavior on the part of Jenna's brother. In the following journal entry she describes both the violence and one of her many reactions to the experience of incest: "If it is important for you to shove a gun up me, poke my breasts, pinch my nipples 'til they bleed, for you to get your anger out, then I am valuable, and therefore I feel important to someone." The incest lasted for three or maybe four years, and ended when her brother went away to college. They are the only two children in a well-to-do professional family, and both were adopted at birth. Jenna says she often "justified" the incest, by telling herself that it was not wrong since they were not really brother and sister. As a child, it never occurred to her to tell anyone, because, as she says, she believed it was her fault. Several years after it stopped she tried to talk about it to a therapist, but it was "brushed off as a natural, exploratory kind of thing," and she says, "I left it at that."

E.B.

E.B. says that when she renamed herself five years ago, it was the first step in a process of empowerment. She refused at first to give me permission to use a pseudonym in this article and had it not been for editorial policy, I would not have done so. "I want to be credited. I want to validate myself. I refuse to give incest power anymore by buying into this silence shit. One reason it continues is because we can't and we won't talk about it. You can't talk about it because you think you did something bad. And you know what? Silence protects the perpetrator. I am not going to be silent anymore." E.B. is a 29 year old white woman, a political activist who has organized an incest survivors' support group. Just a few years ago, like Jenna, her incest was still a secret.

The first thing I remember is playing in a field down the road, and there was a whole gang of us kids. My brother, who is two years older than I am, pulled out a jack-knife saying, "Pull down your pants or I'm gonna stick you." There was tall grass and we were small kids, and somebody got scared and ran and got his mother, and the kids all scattered as soon as they saw her coming. And here I am, a four year old, with my pants around my ankles, and I couldn't go anywhere. And I'm the one that got the shit for it. It was one of the earliest lessons I learned. Don't tell anyone because I'm the one who'll get in trouble. I remember being blamed and feeling terrified.

The really active phase that I remember took place between the ages of 8 and 16, a long time. It included intercourse very early, when I was 9 or 10. When I was 10 we moved from a rural town to a residential neighborhood in a slightly larger town, and I remember hoping it would stop. Now we were going to start a new life, and it was going to be better. But it wasn't.

My brother had his own room. I shared mine with my sister, who is six years younger than I. I remember having to fuck a lot. Sometimes he would grab my arm, twist it up behind my back, and say, "C'mon, we're going for a walk." And we'd go for a walk: out of the yard, up the street, and across the railroad track. Or there was another place down the other way. At some point he began to bring his friends along, and I had to fuck'em all.

My brother and my parents were the only ones who had keys to their bedrooms. My sister and I didn't. Sometimes he would say, "C'mon in and watch TV," or "listen to the stereo." So I would think okay, maybe this time we really can just watch TV. We'd go in, he'd lock the door. Sometimes I'd say no and get physically hurt. Often we'd begin by cuddling, and then go on from there, and there was never the right place to stop. It's like each thing was not so much worse than the thing before. Sometimes it would start by his asking me rub his back, or sometimes he would read aloud to me a passage from an "adult" book, and he'd want to re-enact the same scenario. Sometimes the scenario was rape. Sometimes there was no scenario; it was just plain rape.

About the only thing I got out of it was affection. It was virtually the only affection and intimacy that I had in my life. And there was some affection. Had I to give percentages, I'd say about 80% coercion and physical abuse, and 20% affection. If your only alternative is 1% affection, 20% looks pretty good.

There was a survival strategy I used for getting through it, a fantasy. My brother was very popular, and handsome. The fantasy was that we really loved each other, and if we just weren't brother and sister, may be we'd really be going out. I needed to believe there was at least some love and affection there in order to justify being used.

It stopped when he was 16 and started dating. When he was 18 he went into the Navy. I never talked about it, and I never let people be close to me because I knew that if they really knew what I was, they'd be horrified. I tried to commit suicide twice before I was 18. I was very hurt, very alone, not even safe in my own house. I did well in school, real well, to make up for this hollow place.

I don't know whether my parents knew about the incest at the time. I suspect they do now, but it's something they don't want to confront, don't want to talk about. Three years ago I told them I wouldn't come to the house any time my brother was there, and they have never asked why.

E.B. is a Lesbian. Some authors (e.g., Meiselman, 1978) have suggested a possible connection betweem childhood sexual trauma and later homosexuality, but there is no firm agreement and little research. E.B.'s opinion is that her sexual orientation is unrelated to the incest. "For me," she says, "it feels more like a positive choice than a negative reaction to a traumatic experience."

Discussion

Each of these cases departs in important ways from the accepted view of sibling incest. E.B. and her brother are only two years apart, contrary to the accepted belief that a large age discrepancy is a necessary condition for trauma. Over the past several years I have met other women as well who reported negative experiences with brothers just one or two years older than themselves. Jenna's brother was physically abusive despite the prevailing contention that physical abuse is rare in sibling incest. Another example of physical force comes from Mary, who was abused, sometimes by more than one at the same time, by 3 of her 4 older brothers. They are 1, 8, and 10 years older than she.

> I must have been 7 or so, because we were in the new house. My brother, who I think was 15, told me that from doing the things that we had been doing I could get pregnant, and that was a terrible thing. He said the way to find out was to use this test, which was one of my mother's tampons. I remember his lying me down on the bathroom floor, trying to insert a tampon into my vagina. It was extremely pain- ful, it was just terrible. I was angry at him because it hurt, and I was trying to get him to stop, and he said we have to find out if you're pregnant or not, and so he kept forcing it into me. After that I remember being terribly anxious that maybe I was pregnant, waiting at any moment to start to get big. I don't know for how long I was in pain, but it would hurt a lot if I would urinate.

Current research, not specifically incest-related, indicates that violence among siblings is the most common form of family violence (Straus, et al., 1979), and it is not difficult to imagine the implications for incest between siblings. The research in this area is so sparse that at this point one can only speculate and raise questions for further consideration.

In other significant ways, as well, Jenna's and E.B.'s experiences are characteristic of those I have heard from other women who have been victims of sibling incest. Both women believed that the incest was their fault. Jenna still thinks it was. Both suffered tremendous amounts of guilt. Both knew they would not be believed if they told. Both grew up to struggle with issues of intimacy, self-esteem, and trust. Jenna, as a young adult, has many unresolved sexual difficulties. It is not atypical that E.B.'s brother brought his friends along. If E.B. or Jenna had more than one older brother, it is possible that they, too, like Mary, would have been ganged up on. Judith

Herman (1982) has worked with victims of sibling incest as well as father-daughter incest, and agrees: "Often older brothers gang up or bring in their friends."

Both brothers used bribery and coercion, ingredients present in every instance of sibling incest that has come to my attention. "If you don't do what I ask I'm gonna tell on you," is virtually universal. Both women experienced strong feelings of hurt and anger, and both acknowledged that they derived some gratification from the incest, particularly attention and affection. It is important, however, to examine the component of the gratification that E.B. calls a "survival strategy." Another sibling incest victim uses the same term: "I know there was something I got out of it. I hesitate to say that, because my fear is that I'll be seen as having set it up, and then it becomes my fault. But no matter how horrible something is, you have to figure out something positive you're getting out of it, simply in order to survive. It's a survival strategy." Another sibling incest victim uses the same term: "I know there was something I got out of it. I hesitate to say that, because my fear is that I'll be seen as having set it up, and then it becomes my fault. But no matter how horrible something is, you have to figure out something positive you're getting out of it, simply in order to survive. It's a survival strategy." E.B.'s dating fantasy provided her with the will to survive a situation from which she could not escape, and that otherwise would have been totally intolerable. Jenna's letter to her brother indicates the extreme lengths to which some victims have to go to make such an abhorrent situation tolerable, even valuable.

A legitimate question is why were they unable to stop it? The answer has to do with power. Jenna and E.B. and Mary were younger, and physically smaller than their brothers. Above all, they were girls. Simone de Beauvoir (1952) and Robin Morgan (1978) write about gender-related "demands and rewards" that begin at birth. Girls and boys are not treated the same. Jenna and E.B. describe privileges that were extended to their brothers but not to them. Mary describes it a little differently:

> I was raised in a large Catholic family. The boys were more important than the girls. They were more valued. It was pretty much ingrained in us that my sisters and I and our mother were there to serve them. It never mattered what I felt. Their feelings are what mattered. My feelings don't count at all. Even though one of my brothers was only a year older than I, and I was smarter and better than him in school, I couldn't refuse. I felt too intimidated, too powerless, because he was a boy, because he was taller. I felt like I just had to go along with it.

"Positive" Incest

I have read about instances of "positive" incest, particularly between siblings (e.g., Constantine, 1980). David Finklehor (1980) discusses this issue at some length in his article "Sex Among Siblings," in which he examines the 221 cases of sibling incest that emerged from his larger survey (Finklehor, 1979). He states that "reactions to the experiences were equally divided among those who considered them positively and negatively." The question of positive and negative requires close inspection. Although the reactions were mixed, it is significant that in the younger-sister older-brother category, the sisters more often reported negative reactions and the brothers more often reported positive reactions.

But what of the sisters whose reactions were positive? What does the term positive mean to them? Finklehor's findings, based almost entirely on a written questionnaire, offer no further information. Possibly their relationships with their brothers were egalitarian. Possibly their sex was a caring give and take. Possibly they initiated equally, and neither was receiving pleasure at the other's expense. But I have not encountered such a sibling sexual relationship.

More likely, they had been trained, like Mary, to put another's pleasure before their own, and derived satisfaction from "doing their duty." This kind of girl or woman might value herself in relation to how valued she is by an older male, in this case her brother. This is clearly related to the "survival strategy" described by both Jenna and E.B. of finding a positive side to the horror. Or perhaps the explanation lies in what Carlos Laredo (1982) calls "denial of impact." "An interesting clinical note," he says, "is that once sibling incest was uncovered or revealed, many clients indicated no difficulties resulting from the incest. This outcome was belied by underlying dynamics of conflict, confusion, or guilt that were identified by the clinician. . . . For many of these same adult clients, unresolved conflicts resulting from sibling incest were major therapeutic issues, nevertheless." An example from a co-therapy team is "C" (Silberman, 1981), who at 9 or 10 became involved in an incestuous relationship with her 11 year old brother. "The relationship progressed to intercourse by age 12. C. reports never being coerced, having positive sexual feelings, and eventually orgasm." Her therapists go on to say that now, at the age of 21, she is unable to have intercourse with her husband, and has a phobic aversion to sex.

Several authors (Butler, 1978; Herman, 1981; Rush, 1980; Sanford, 1980) point out that incest by mutual consent is psychologically impossible when the participants are unequal in power. Therefore, they say, parent-child sex is necessarily exploitative. This may be equally true for sex between an older brother and a younger sister.

Recuperation*

Even when the victim perceives the incest as benign, the aftereffects suggest it is not. They include—for survivors of all types of incest—depression and suicide attempts, drug-addiction, low self-esteem, repeated victimization, lack of assertiveness, sexual dysfunction, migraine headaches, intense distrust of others, difficulty establishing and maintaining long-term relationships, and confusion between intimacy and sexuality.

The first step on the road from victim to survivor is hearing from friends, therapists, other survivors, that it was not her fault, that she was not powerful enough to stop it, and that her powerlessness was not her fault either. The survivor of sibling incest may need to hear this many times. She may have internalized the myth that sibling sex is benign, and then feel confused and invalidated because she does not experience it that way. In other respects, she needs what all incest survivors need: the opportunity to tell her story, at her own pace; to identify and express her anger and the rest of the complex tangle of emotions that she feels; to understand the relationship between the incest and its aftereffects; to meet with other survivors and learn that she is not alone. Recuperation can be slow and difficult, but it is possible. Survivors can deal with the pain, trauma, and anger, and go on to live satisfying lives.

For E.B. the important parts were going public (writing newspaper articles, speaking out), organizing and participating in a survivors' support group, and, later, confronting her brother in a strongly worded letter with his crime and her rage. Mary, too, found that a peer support group worked for her. She says, "By talking with other survivors I came to understand that the powerlessness and hopelessness I felt as an adult stemmed from the same feelings that I experienced as a child at the hands of my brothers." Jenna is in a different place. For her to share her journal was a big first step. Perhaps next she will be able to talk directly to a therapist, preferably one with a feminist orientation who will understand the dynamics of victimization. Eventually she may contact other survivors, perhaps beginning with books rather than real people.

---

*Thanks to Mellen Kennedy, a Montpelier, Vermont counselor, for suggesting this term.

Prevention

The perpetuation of incest depends in the short run on the silence of the victim. E.B. prevents incest when she refuses to protect the aggressor. Judith Herman (1981) proposes sex education that begins early in grade school, to present basic information on sexuality and sexual assault. Linda Sanford (1980) has written a parents' guide connecting the prevention of child sexual abuse and the self-esteem enhancement of children.

In the long run, incest will stop when males, of *any* age, are no longer more powerful and more privileged than females, when females, of *any* age, are confident and empowered to say no. Ultimately, harmful sibling incest will stop when there is a transformation of our male-defined society, when "little girls are brought up from the first with the same demands and rewards, the same severity and the same freedom, as her brothers . . ." (de Beauvoir, 1952).

Summary

This article has discussed incest between older brothers and younger sisters within a social context. The relationship between big brothers and little sisters contains many of the same elements as relationships between fathers and daughters, and husbands and wives. Reports of positive sibling incest should be carefully examined. Sibling incest can be, and often is, as traumatizing as sexual abuse of a child by an adult.

REFERENCES

Beauvoir, S. de. *The Second Sex*. Trans. and ed. by H. M. Parshley. New York: Alfred A. Knopf, 1952.

Butler, S. *Conspiracy of Silence: The Trauma of Incest*. San Francisco: New Glide Publications, 1978.

Constantine, L. "Effects of Early Sexual Experiences: A Review and Synthesis of Research," in L. L. Constantine and F. M. Martinson, *Children and Sex: New Findings, New Perspectives*. Boston: Little, Brown, 1980

Finklehor, D. "Sex Among Siblings: A Survey Report on its Prevalence, Its Variety and Its Effects." *Archives of Sexual Behavior* 9 (1980): pp. 171–194.

Finklehor, D. *Sexually Victimized Children*. New York: Free Press, 1979.

Forward, S. and Buck, C. *Betrayal of Innocence: Incest and its Devastation*. Los Angeles: J. P. Tarcher, 1978.

Francoeur, R. *Becoming a Sexual Person*. New York: John Wiley and Sons, 1982.

Good, J. "Coping with Incest." *The Vermont Vanguard Press* 4 (March 6–13, 1981): pp. 10–11.

Herman, J. *Father-Daughter Incest*. Cambridge, Mass.: Harvard Univ. Press, 1981.

Herman, J. personal communication, March 7, 1982.

Justice, B. and Justice, R. *The Broken Taboo: Sex in the Family*. New York: Human Science Press, 1979.

Laredo, C. "Sibling Incest." In S. M. Sgroi, ed. *Handbook of Clinical Intervention in Child Sexual Abuse*. Lexington, Mass.: Heath and Co., 1982, pp. 177–188.

Lester, D. "Incest." *J. of Sex Research* 8 (1972): pp. 268–285.

Lukianowicz, N. "Incest II: Other Types of Incest." *British J. of Psychiatry* 120 (1972): pp. 308–313.

Meiselman, K. *Incest: A Psychological Study of Causes and Effects with Treatment Recommendations*. San Francisco: Jossey-Bass, 1978.

Morgan, R. *Going Too Far: The Personal Chronicle of a Feminist*. New York: Vintage Books, 1978.

Rush, F. *Best Kept Secret: Sexual Abuse of Children*. Englewood Cliffs, N.J.: Prentice-Hall, 1980.

Sanford, L. *The Silent Children: A Parents' Guide to the Prevention of Child Sexual Abuse*. New York: Doubleday Anchor Press, 1980.

Silberman, G. and Silberman, L. "Case History: Phobic Avoidance of Sex." Unpublished ms., 1981.

Straus, M., Gelles, R., and Steinmetz, S. *Behind Closed Doors: Violence in the American Family*. New York: Doubleday, 1979.

Strong, B. and Reynolds, R. *Understanding Our Sexuality*. St. Paul, Minn.: West Publ. Co., 1982.

Weeks, R. "The Sexually Exploited Child." *Southern Medical J.* 69, 7 (1976): pp. 848–850.

A STUDY OF ISSUES
IN SEXUALITY COUNSELING FOR WOMEN
WITH SPINAL CORD INJURIES

Janna Zwerner

Introduction

Disabled consumers have made the demand for social and physical integration into the mainstream of contemporary life. This rise of consumer awareness has opened up a Pandora's box for professionals working in the disabled community. Not only are there psychological and vocational issues to face, there are social and sexual issues as well. Until recently, the sexual needs of individuals with physical disabilities has been largely ignored by the rehabilitation community and not recognized as an area of legitimate concern for social service professionals. In particular, little information is available concerning the sexual functioning of spinal cord injured women.

The sexual problems of disabled women in general stem from two sources: those resulting from cultural myths and attitudinal barriers, and those resulting from actual physical limitations. We are all subjected to societal mandates encouraging romantic and spontaneous sexual relations, and sexual intercourse and orgasm are often seen as crucial for sexual fulfillment. Such rules are harmful to us all, but particularly so to disabled people. These assumptions about sex may lead to a sense of failure for disabled women, interfering with the realization that sexuality is not limited to a specific act. "When these beliefs are recognized as myths by the individuals, the problems arise from physical limitations seem much less formidable."[1]

Traditional public sentiment has stigmatized the disabled as being asexual, or at best, undesirable dating and sexual partners. For many years, the use of sublimation was advocated as an effective and final technique for dealing with sexual impulses.[2] Many individuals, including physicians and rehabilitation practitioners, still hold the belief that after being confined to a wheelchair one's sexual life was over.[3]

Janna Zwerner is a rehabilitation counselor and consultant specializing in the field of sexuality and disabled women. She is currently Director of Services at Boston Self Help Center.

91

Review of the Literature

It has only been since 1972 that rehabilitation literature has considered sexuality as integral to the total psychological adjustment to disability.[4] While references are available in specialized medical journals concerning specific disabilities and their sexual concomitants, this information has not been brought to the attention of social service practitioners, and has received little attention in rehabilitation journals.[5]

Information concerning the sexual functioning of spinal cord injured (SCI) males is in abundance relative to the literature pertaining to SCI females. This discrepancy is partially due to the fact that 4 out of every 5 SCI individuals are males.[6] However, the attitude exists that sexual problems are not as traumatic for the SCI woman because she usually "plays the passive role in sexual relations."[7] This is also assumed to be the case because almost all SCI women continue to remain fertile. Thus, the sexual functioning of SCI females have not had the same level of serious inquiry as compared to studies of SCI males.

Physiological Considerations

As early as 1917, Riddoch[8] reported on the sexual response of paraplegic men with complete and incomplete spinal lesions. Since then, numerous studies have produced detailed information, classified according to the level and completeness of the lesion, coupled with a "statistical prognosis" of the probability of reflexogenic sexual response in males.[9,10] However, very little similar descriptive data is available on the physiological and psychogenic aspects of sexual response in women with lesions at various levels.[11] Griffith and Trieschmann[12] postulated the presence of a "genital reflex" in SCI women paralleling the reflex found in SCI men. The functions involved in this reflexogenic response would include vascular engorgement of the clitoris, labia minora and vagina, and increased secretions of the Bartholin glands. Nevertheless, clinical observations are scarce, and comprehensive research with SCI women is still severely lacking.

The large majority of reports that do exist concentrate on the reproductive aspect of female sexuality, that is, menstruation, fertility, and pregnancy.[13,14] There appears to be great intrigue with SCI women's reproductive ability, most likely because their male conterparts often quickly become infertile. Many SCI women also go through a painless labor process, providing a unique phenomenon to study for the medical community. Yet, there is an increased risk of autonomic dysreflexia,* post-partum uterine prolapse, and susceptibility to infection. In some cases this preoccupation with the childbearing capacity of SCI women has led to the erroneous belief that "woman patients have no loss of physical sexual function."[16] Crigler[17] suggested that this assumption may be due to the fact that erectile and ejaculatory functions are often impaired in men, whereas "sexual dysfunction is not as graphically apparent in an injured woman." Even if this suggestion were true, one cannot forget that for a large segment of our society, women's sexuality exists for the sole purpose of perpetuating our species, bereft of satisfaction, except for pleasing one's spouse and creating offspring. Furthermore, it is difficult to imagine that a SCI woman would consider her own "sexual dysfunction [as not] graphically apparent."

A few studies noted disturbances in the orgasmic phase of female sexual response.[9,18] When spinal lesions were complete, women were often "anorgasmic," but were sexually aroused by intense tactile stimulation above the sensory level, especially around the breasts.[12] In many instances there is an overly sensitive zone above the level of injury, also heightened in an erogenous sense. It is evident in numerous subjective reports of both paraplegic and quadriplegic women that erotogenic areas may be found in places where they previously had produced little or no sexual excitement.[19,20]

A wide variety of experiences were interpreted as orgasm and usually involved muscle contraction and spasticity followed by a generalized decrease in muscle tension.[12,20] Peripheral responses to sexual stimulation, such as increased respiration and blood pressure, swelling of the breasts, and a sex flush, often remained intact.[21] Money[22,23] reported the experience of "phantom orgasm" in the dreams and waking imagery of paraplegic men and women who did not have voluntary movement or somatic sensation in the genito-pelvic area. The use of the word "phantom" is questionable at best, and at worst, downright oppressive to the disabled individual. Nongenitally based orgasms are possible and it seems senseless to demean the complex experience of climax as being "phantom." These findings underscore the subjective interpretation of orgasm, giving clinical foundation to the wide variety of sexual response in humans. This holds particularly true for the female orgasmic experience which displays greater diversification in the intensity and duration of response than the male's relatively standard pattern of ejaculatory reaction.[24]

---

*This condition causes a rapid increase in blood pressure, profuse sweating and flushing, and a pounding headache. It occurs in injuries about the T4-T6 level, and can be fatal if not brought under rapid control.[15]

Previous research defined libido as interest in sexual intercourse and focused on the act of coitus as the predominant mode of sexual interaction.[18,25] But the common notion of "the sex act" (male superior position) as the foundation of sexual intimacy is no longer a valid concept for many individuals, and particularly for severely disabled women. An increased risk toward urinary and vaginal infections, spasms, lack of lubrication and sensation, and personal preferences may make intercourse undesirable to many SCI women. None of these reasons necessarily dampen sexual drives nor rid one of the reality of sexual being. Thus, it is not surprising that many studies reported a marked decrease in sexual activities (intercourse) amongst many physically disabled populations.[25] This appears crucial in light of recent research with SCI couples showing that those with a greater acceptance of sexual variety tended to be more satisfied with their sexual activities. It was speculated that other couples had a higher tolerance for less sexual activity due to a lack of adequate information about their sexuality.[26]

Often, it is simply the facts that are needed to dispel myths and thorough information dissemination becomes of the utmost importance. After interviewing 19 SCI women, Becker[27] found those with the most accurate and extensive information regarding their sexuality have fewer emotional conflicts emerging from sexual conflicts. These findings support the need for information and sexuality counseling designed to increase sexual repertoire and acceptance of sexual variety. Sexuality counseling should also include a basic explanation of spinal cord physiology in order to promote an understanding of post-injury sexual response.

Psychosocial Considerations

In some circumstances the emotional sequelae of a new physical disability may interfere with sexual functioning. Traumatic SCI affects a person in a myriad of ways, not only neurologically, but psychologically and socially as well. Wright has suggested that because "sex identification is often a central personal characteristic that serves to define the person to herself and others, it can be expected that any circumstance that alters or endangers this identification will have a marked effect on the self concept."[28] Self concept is known to influence sexual attitudes and activities, just as sexual adjustment will play a role in defining and enhancing self concept.[29]

Teal and Athelstan[30] reviewed numerous articles investigating changes in self concept through their expression in changed body image. The total experience of one's body image is resistant to abrupt modification and some authors noted a tendency to maintain a pre-injury body image, with more difficulty in body image adjustment for quadriplegics than paraplegics. However, very few of the studies reviewed included female subjects in their samples. Rather, post-injury feelings of feminine attractiveness has more frequently been studied in SCI women. Perhaps not surprisingly, many aspects of femininity and attractiveness are the same for SCI women as they are for non-disabled women.[31,32] Yet, many women stressed that although they were currently involved in sexual relationships and had a positive self image, the first few years after injury were extremely difficult. Most of the women mentioned a lack of understanding and sensitivity by health professionals of their sexual needs and viewed this as a hindrance in adjustment to their disability.

It is not uncommon for individuals to experience depression, lowered self esteem, changed self image, or performance fears as a result of stress at the time of injury. A trained counselor can provide emotional support and assistance in working through these feelings. Thornton[33] revealed that in her work with SCI women, brief therapy, initiated for emotional problems related to sexual expression, was often very successful. Important areas in sexuality counseling were outlined, including learning one's current sexual response and sexual experimentation. Although it had been believed that a great deal of practice over a long period of time was essential to a fulfilling sex life among the cord injured, little correlation was found between sexual adjustment and time since injury.[34]

Perhaps the belief that SCI males go through a more difficult sexual identity readjustment process has contributed to the lack of research regarding women in this area. Several of the reports endorsing this notion were published in the late 60s and early 70s. While these beliefs may have held true for some women at that time, they are most definitely rapidly changing in the present. In an era where exploration of non-traditional social and vocational roles are being encouraged for women, these assumptions uphold traditional sex role stereotypes and attitudinal barriers regarding disabled women. Despite the recent emphasis on sexual concerns in the severely disabled, many health care and social service practitioners remain uninformed of available resources and indifferent to the special needs of their female clients. "I shall end by asking whether the increasing awareness of sexual problems of the disabled is no more than a facade? What is really being done and for whom?"[35]

Methodology

An information packet describing the study was mailed to over 50 SCI treatment and counseling centers. Fourteen geographically dispersed agencies participated and distributed 170 questionnaires to SCI women who were at least one month but no more than 7 years post-injury. The self administered anonymous questionnaire was returned by 88 women, but only 68 were usable following the above criteria.

The questionnaire was designed to assess the quality and perceived need for sexuality counseling services offered by social service and health care professionals. There were 21 questions requiring approximately thirty minutes to complete. With respect to the philosophy of self help and consumer concern, respondents were encouraged to list the kinds of services and information they viewed as imperative to post-injury sexuality counseling. Due to the limitations of space and the specific focus of this report, a more detailed analysis will not be presented here.

Results and Discussion

Out of the 68 participants who participated in this study, only 30 (44%) received some type of sexuality counseling. These women were asked to rate the quality of their session(s) on 15 different items for both emotional counseling and informational content. A four point scale was used as follows:

1. No counseling or information (The topic was not mentioned).
2. Fair counseling or information (Feelings and attitudes, or some facts about the topic were briefly mentioned).
3. Good counseling or information (Feelings and attitudes, or some facts and details about the topic were discussed in general terms).
4. Excellent counseling or information (Feelings and attitudes, or facts and details were thoroughly discussed in personal terms, including options or alternatives for you).

Overall, the informational content was only slightly better than the counseling content, although this varied widely from topic to topic. The mean quality on the informational scale was 2.32, with only 13 (44.8%) of the 30 women scoring a "4" for any one topic. The most information was received on topics such as physical sexual functioning, sexual/sensual sensations, and bladder and bowel control. The least information was given on topics such as lesbianism, sexual aids, and masturbation. Rather, information dissemination centered around issues related to sexual functioning and performance, as opposed to a focus directed toward sexual exploration and education. Items designed to increase sexual repertoire and acceptance of alternative modes of sexual expression could have been emphasized much more. All participants indicated a far greater need for more information than they received, and there was no one area where the desire for information was matched or surpassed by the information received. The topics notably lacking in this area were sexual complications related to disability, sexual positions, birth control methods and their side effects, and orgasm.

Perhaps not surprisingly, participants wanted access to more information than they had been given. There has traditionally been a tremendous amount of confusion surrounding female sexuality and only recently has the vaginal vs. clitoral orgasm been resolved. Furthermore, several reports[26,27] suggest that the more accurate information one has regarding sexuality, the less dissatisfaction and emotional problems one will have in sexual adjustment. It seems likely that the heightened interest in such topics as sexual complications related to disability, birth control methods, and orgasm, probably reflect a lack of knowledge and available information regarding the sexual functioning of SCI women, emphasizing the need for extensive research in this area.

In contrast, the mean quality on the emotional counseling scale was 2.26, with only 10 (33.3%) women scoring a "4" for any one topic. Once again counseling centered around items related to sexual functioning and performance. Sexual morality and sexual positions were not mentioned in 13 of the 30 cases, and masturbation and sexual aids were not mentioned in 16 and 18 cases, respectively.

In a few areas, counseling received actually exceeded the perceived need for this service. For example, considerably more counseling was given than desired on the topic of bladder and bowel control. It has long been believed that incontinence poses a major problem for SCI persons in sexual relations, this being stressed in many of the books and articles reviewed in this study. The findings here tend to support those of Bregman[32] who reported that although women found bladder and bowel problems an inconvenience, it was not felt to be a serious problem interfering with their sexual experiences.*

The issues viewed as most important to the counseling dimension were psycho-social and -sexual in nature. For example, participants desired more counseling on topics such as their sexuality, partners, and other's view of

---

*A regular bladder and bowel program can greatly reduce the risk of "accidents." There are many options here which should be openly discussed between sexual partners. See reference #20.

their sexuality. Many women were specific in stating their needs and interests in these areas, especially regarding the development of social skills necessary to obtain partners and form intimate relationships. A lack of sexual partners has been cited as a major reason for dissatisfaction with sexual activity in disabled individuals.[36] Assertiveness has been suggested as a partial remedy to this problem, being an important precondition in satisfactory adaptation to traumatic injury.[37] When carried over to the sexual realm of one's life, assertiveness enhanced interpersonal relationships and communication during sex. Increasing communication skills in social situations will often provide for the confidence and feedback necessary to venture out and meet potential partners, thereby intensifying one's desirability. It might be advantageous to include elements of assertiveness training in post-injury counseling programs to help overcome fears of rejection and counteract assumptions that SCI woman are or want to be passive. Furthermore, this skill seems crucial for disabled women requiring special preparation and assistance in order to ready themselves for lovemaking.

In terms of general sexuality counseling one might expect the focus to be the client's understanding of her own sexuality, given the basic goal of exploration of feelings and values, and increased self awareness. It would not be expected that the topic of lesbianism would be thoroughly discussed unless the client was a lesbian or bisexual (only 6 in the total sample fell into these categories). However, masturbation would be a concern for all women, particularly those adjusting to an altered body image and physical sensations, yet this item received almost no attention on both the informational and counseling scales. Also infrequently mentioned were other items designed to increase acceptance of sexual variety, such as sexual aids and sexual positions. It appears that the taboo on discussing explicit sexual acts remained intact during many of the counseling sessions.

A newly injured woman may need permission to explore and reaffirm her sexuality. Each injury and individual will be different, and clients should be encouraged to find the solutions that work best for them. Just as sexual response will vary widely in women who are not disabled, this will also hold true for SCI women, even with injuries at about the same level. Reluctance on behalf of the counselor to bring up topics such as self pleasuring, oral sex, and the use of sexual aids tends to discourage sexual experimentation. It might prove beneficial to keep in mind that not too long ago the client was not disabled, and may very well have held some misconceptions about the sexual lives of disabled persons.

Summary

Despite the increasing awareness of the sexual needs of disabled individuals, less than half of the participants in this study received some type of sexuality counseling as a result of their injury. Many of the women who did receive services were dissatisfied with their counseling sessions and the lack of available information regarding their sexuality. It is hoped that in the near future sexuality counseling will become an integral part of the rehabilitation process, and that disabled women will have the same access to information about their sexuality as do their male counterparts.

REFERENCES

1. Saxton, M. A peer counseling training program for disabled women. *Journal of Sociology and Social Welfare*, September, 1981.

2. Holbert, D. A. Sex and the disabled. *Rehabilitation Gazette*, 19: 14–15, 1967.

3. Wada, M. A., Brodwin, M. G. Attitudes of society toward sexual functioning of male individuals with spinal cord injuries. *Psychology*, 12(4), 18–22, 1975.

4. Kaplan, S. Sexual counseling for persons with spinal cord injuries: A literature review. *Journal of Applied Rehabilitation Counseling*, 10(4), 200–203, 1979.

5. Cole, T. M., Glass, D. D. Commentary: Sexuality and physical disabilities. *Archives of Physical Medicine and Rehabilitation*, 58(12), 585–586, 1977.

6. Young, J. S. National Spinal Cord Injury Data Research Center. Personal communication, 1980.

7. Singh, S. P., Magner, T. Sex and the self: The spinal cord injured. *Rehabilitation Literature*, 36(1), 2–10, 1975.

8. Riddoch, G. The reflex function of the completely divided spinal cord in man, compared with those associated with less severe lesions. *Brain*, 40: 264–402, 1917.

9. Heslings, K., Scheller, A. M., Verkuyl, A. Not Made of Stone: The Sexual Problems Of Handicapped People. Springfield, Illinois: Charles C. Thomas, 1974.

10. Comarr, A. E. Sex classifications and expectations among quadriplegics and paraplegics. *Sexuality and Disability*, 1(4), 252–259, 1978.

11. Geiger, R. C. Neurophysiology of sexual response in spinal cord injury. *Sexuality and Disability*, 2(4), 257–266, 1979.

12. Griffith, E. R., Trieschmann, R. B. Sexual functioning in women with spinal cord injury. *Archives of Physical Medicine and Rehabilitation*, 56(1), 18–21, 1975.

13. Comarr, A. E. Observations on menstruation and pregnancy among female spinal cord injury patients. *Paraplegia*, 3: 263–271, 1966.

14. Robertson, D. N. S. Pregnancy and labor in the paraplegic. *Paraplegia*, 10: 209–212, 1972.

15. Erickson, R. P. Autonomic hyperreflexia: Pathophysiology and medical management. *Archives of Physical Medicine and Rehabilitation*, 61: 431–440, 1980.

16. Coleman, N. J. Sexual information in the rehabilitation process. *Journal of Applied Rehabilitation Counseling*, 5(1), 201–206, 1974.

17. Crigler, L. Sexual concerns of the spinal cord injured. *Nursing Clinics of North America*, 9(4), 703–717, 1974.

18. Griffith, E. R., Tomko, M. A., Timms, R. J. Sexual function in spinal cord injured patients: A review. *Archives of Physical Medicine and Rehabilitation*, 54(12), 539–543, 1973.

19. Becker, E. F. Female Sexuality Following Spinal Cord Injury, Bloomington, Illinois: Accent press, 1978.

20. Shaul, S., Bogle, J., Harbaugh, J. H., Norman, A. D. Toward Intimacy: Family Planning and Sexuality Concerns of Physically Disabled Women. New York: Human Sciences Press, 1980.

21. Cole, T. M. Sexuality and physical disabilities. *Archives of Sexual Behavior*, 4(4), 389–403, 1975.

22. Money, J. Phantom orgasm in the dreams of paraplegic men and women. *Archives of General Psychiatry*, 3: 373–382, 1960.

23. Money, J. Phantom orgasm in paraplegics. *Medical Aspects in Human Sexuality*, 4(1), 90–99, 1970.

24. Master, W. H., Johnson, V. E. Human Sexual Response. Boston: Little, Brown and Co., 1966.

25. Ferro, J. M., Allen, H. A. Sexuality: The effects of physical impairment. *Rehabilitation Counseling Bulletin*, 20(2), 148–151, 1976.

26. Steger, J. C., Brockway, J. A. Sexual enhancement in spinal cord injured patients: Behavioral group treatment. *Sexuality and Disability*, 3(2), 84–96, 1980.

27. Becker, E. F. Sexuality and the spinal cord injured woman: An interview. *Sexuality and Disability*, 2(4), 278–286, 1979.

28. Wright, B. A. Physical Disability: A Psychological Approach. New York: Harper and Row, 1960.

29. Romano, M. Sexuality and the disabled female. *Sexuality and Disability*, 1(1), 27–33, 1978.

30. Teal, J. C., Athelstan, G. T. Sexuality and spinal cord injury: Some psychosocial implications. *Archives of Physical Medicine and Rehabilitation*,56(6), 264–268, 1975.

31. Fitting, M. D., Salisbury, S., Davies, N. H., Mayclin, D. K. Self concept and sexuality of spinal cord injured women. *Archives of Sexual Behavior*, 7(2), 143–156, 1978.

32. Bregman, S. Sexual adjustment of spinal cord injured women. *Sexuality and Disability*, 1(2), 85–92, 1978.

33. Thornton, C. E. Sexuality counseling of women with spinal cord injuries. *Sexuality and Disability*, 2(4), 267–277, 1979.

34. Bregman, S., Hadley, R. G. Sexual adjustment and feminine attractiveness among spinal cord injured women. *Archives of Physical Medicine and Rehabilitation*, 57: 448–450, 1976.

35. Nordqvist, I. Sexual counseling for disabled persons. *Sexuality and Disability*, 3(3), 193–198, 1980.

36. Halstead, L. S., Halstead, M. M., Salhoot, J. T., Stock, D. D., Sparks, R. W. A hospital-based program in human sexuality. *Archives of Physical Medicine and Rehabilitation*, 58(9), 409–412, 1977.

37. Dunn, M., Lloyd, E. E., Phelps, G. H. Sexual assertiveness in spinal cord injury. *Sexuality and Disability*, 2(4), 293–306, 1979.

COUNSELING WOMEN WITH DEVELOPMENTAL DISABILITIES

Margaret Downes

In her book, *Toward a New Psychology of Women*, Jean Baker Miller states:

> Women have played a specific role in a male-led society in ways no other suppressed groups have done. They have been entwined with men in intimate and intense relationships, creating the milieu—the family—in which the human mind as we know it has been formed. Thus women's situation is a crucial key to understanding the psychological order.

One could apply this statement to persons with disabilities, that the women's role may be a "crucial key" to defining the role of all disabled persons in our society. The focus of this paper will be on women with developmental disabilities and their counseling needs. The criteria used to define developmental disabilities (commonly referred to as mental retardation) is the three part definition developed by the American Association on Mental Deficiency: 1. significantly subaverage general intellectual functioning: and IQ of 70 or below; 2. concurrent deficits in adaptive behavior; 3. Onset before the age of 18-22. The categories of intellectual impairment are defined as: Mild-IQ between 55–69; Moderate-40 to 54; Severe-25 to 39; and profound-0 to 29 (Hurley & Sovner, 1982).

The purpose of this paper is to offer clinicians insight and increased awareness of the counseling needs of women with developmental disabilities. Thus, gaining a better understanding of the needs of all persons with intellectual impairment and their families.

Margaret Downes is an educator who has specialized in working with Special Needs populations and their families for eleven years.

Methods of Research

The questionnaire-interview method of research was used to collect the information from the subjects discussed in this paper. Each subject was given a copy of the questionnaire which was read to her to insure her understanding of it. The interviews took approximately one and a half hours and were conducted in a place of the subject's choice.

Review and Discussion of the Literature

The following is a review and brief discussion of some of the research over the past decade in the area of developmental disabilities. Included are excerpts from interviews conducted with mental health professionals active in this area.

Why counseling for the women with developmental disabilities? Are the needs of the women of this population special? Approximately 80% of developmental disabilities persons fall into the mild to moderate range. That means that their verbal skills are appropriate to various forms of action and play oriented therapies, as well as the more traditional talk and behavioral therapies. About 85% of all intellectually impaired persons by virtue of their socialization as second class citizens are prone to an anxiety (Menolascino, 1970). According to Miller (1976), women are socialized to a subservient position. One may conclude that women with developmental disabilities are hit with a dual subservience in our society, that of women and that of mentally and intellectually impaired (as the society views it). Studies show that for women present with higher rates of depression than men (Weissman & Klerman, 1977), this dual social barrier carried by women with intellectual impairment (not to mention ethnic and language considerations) must affect a woman's self esteem in one way—negatively.

Abbot and Ladd (1970) state the literature on marriage of persons who have developmental disabilities indicates that they are capable of managing satisfactory marriages. This suggests an increased need for sexual and related areas counseling for this population. In particular, since the responsibility for birth control and child rearing falls to the women in our culture.

Sletten et al. (1972) reported on suicide rates in a mental hospital population. Among the population sample they did report on the suicide rate of persons who are "mentally retarded" but the sample was small and the evidence inconclusive. Interestingly, they identified mental retardation as the psychiatric illness. Whereas recent reports confirm that a person with a developmental disability may develop any of the affective disorders, but developmental disability is not a harbinger of psychiatric disorder. Sovner and Hurley (1982) concluded in their review of reports regarding the occurrence of affective illness in persons with intellectual impairment that "the psychiatrically symptomatic person with MR should always be evaluated for affective symptomatology and be considered for the full range of treatments. . . ." In an interview, Dr. Sovner (3/1/82) expressed concern regarding the use of drugs with this population. He said, "You have people in state facilities or community residences who are on outrageous combinations of drugs. The most common question I am asked is does this person need this drug? My answer is that I don't know, let's take her off the drug and see." Plotkin and Gill label this kind of abuse as "invisible manacles that indicate the societal prejudice prevailing against persons with developmental disabilities" (1978).

There may be different affective symptoms with persons with developmental disabilities than in the general population (Sovner & Hurley, 1980). For example, aggressive acting out, withdrawal, and/or somatic complaints may be observed instead of classic complaints, i.e., feelings of hopelessness.

Dr. Sylvia Scheinkoff, a psychologist and practicing psychotherapist in the greater Boston area, in an interview (3/29/82), spoke of the legal mandate to service this population. For example, de-institutionalization, P.L. 94–142, is causing mental health professionals to look at these "hidden people," who must now be served in different ways. She said, "This is a good thing. Those who have been interested in the needs of this population will continue to be. Others will take an opportunistic stance and see this as something to latch onto, and others will hear about the issue from their professional peers and get another point of view about persons with mental retardation. They will hear and perhaps understand that persons with mental retardation do have a psychological entity within themselves and will begin to think that perhaps there is something there that might enhance them and interest them as clinicians." She continues regarding the type of therapy to use with this population, "When you are a therapist of a person with mental retardation if you are not a creative person, you are not going to hit the mark. . . . If you are locked into a special way of doing things, if you are expecting a lot of help from your patient, you may become a frustrated clinician. Insight develops slowly and not to the degree that it develops in the person who is not retarded."

Smiley (1973) presents a common attitude toward developmentally disabled persons in his article about sterilization. As a rule the mental defect is accompanied by more or less mental instability." Though much is said about abortion and sterilization, the person's ability to make an informed consent about this very important part of her sexuality does not seem to be fully addressed. Further, Sovner and Hurley (1982) state that mental retardation is a level of intelligence and social functioning, not an illness. Persons with developmental disabilities may exhibit symptoms of affective illness; however, in this writer's opinion to imply that "mental instability" is inevitable is inaccurate.

In terms of responsible and healthy birth control for women with developmental disabilities, Bass (1978) presents a reasonable look at surgical contraception. At a time when normalization procedures have persons with intellectual impairment developing an acceptance of themselves and their right to their sexuality, the government is doing a backslide on subsidies for sterilization, birth control and abortions. Some evidence is given by Bass that a great majority of developmentally disabled persons are capable of deciding this step for themselves. He discusses surgical contraception for both men and women and outlines areas for further research.

Certainly, the evidence is present that women with developmental disabilities experience the same second class socialization as women in the general population, i. e., depression, drug abuse and subservience show this. Further, because of their disability, they are very likely to be at greater risk and have less intellectual resources available to gain therapeutic and educational support.

Subjects and Responses to the Questionnaire

Subject 1. C. is a 25 year old woman who is living independently in the community. She is presently living with a man friend and they have been sharing their apartment with her parents and brother. C. and her friend have decided to get a place of their own. C. spent a good deal of her adolescence in a foster home, her family of origin being alcoholic. It is not clear why she has reconnected with them at this time. She attended special education classes in a public school system through the junior high level and then went to a vocational training school for the developmentally disabled. C.'s disability appears to be mild.

Subject 2. H. is an eighteen year old woman who lives with her mother, brother (older) and three younger siblings. Her brother is about 24 and the other siblings are adolescents. Father is not in the home and it is not clear for how long but he is now living out of state. The family is strongly Irish Catholic. H. attends a public school special education program where she was interviewed. H. appears to be moderately disabled, though her verbal skills seem poor it is not clear if it is intellectual in nature or emotional. She exhibits inappropriate behavior for her age and both the school and home have "complained" of her masturbating in front of people. Her mother's reaction is to punish her, the school personnel, fearful of parent complaint, have tried to be neutral. The school and family both have complained of acting out behavior on H.'s part.

Subject 3. D. is a thirty-nine year old woman who lives in a cottage home setting in a state institution. D. seems to be a very angry person as is manifested in contortions of her facial features during conversation, body language (she sits with arms and legs tightly entwined and turned away from the interviewer) and verbal expressions of anger. Her family of origin was large and Irish Catholic though it is not clear how much contact she has with them now. D.'s main interpersonal relationships are with the staff of the cottage, who have a difficult time tolerating her sour personality. D. grew frustrated with the questionnaire after a short time and kept trying to bring the conversation around to her last episode of running away. D. appears to have a low moderate disability.

For the purposes of this paper the author has narrowed her concerns to the following areas within the questionnaire:

1. Reaction to questions regarding sex and knowledge of their own sexuality and that of their partner, interest in more information.
2. Has or is sex been or being discussed in a therapy or educational setting and who initiated it?
3. Has the subject ever felt as if she could not go on, felt hopeless or felt like killing herself?
4. The state of the subject's present interpersonal relationships with people of both sexes.

C.'s response to question 1 indicated she definitely was interested in more information about her own sexuality and that of her partner. Though embarrassed at first, she readily agreed that she was confused about birth control, pregnancy and the reading material the vocational school had given her about sex. When the interviewer asked what she had done with the material she replied that she still had it but could not read it! She also expressed interest in better understanding orgasm, masturbation (which when explained to her, she had never heard of or done), pregnancy and marriage (since she did hope to marry one day and have children). C. had been in therapy following hospitalization for a suicide attempt (she tried to walk through a glass door, jump out a window) four years ago and has continued to see her therapist though no longer wants to kill herself. She has never discussed her concerns regarding sex with her therapist. For socialization she and her partner visit with other couples and C. visits with neighbors during the day. She says she gets a lot out of the relationship, he takes care of the money and she runs the house, but she would like to marry him however he claims he is too old for her (a 14 year age difference). She would like a job but has had difficulty finding one since finishing school.

Issues: C. needs education regarding physical and emotional aspects of male and female sexuality.

—needs to develop sense of own self-worth separate from her partner, also career counseling would help her gain this and contribute to family finances.

Clinician's Role: help C. get information regarding her own and partner's sexuality, perhaps a group workshop type program in which she could gain some self confidence as well as sex education.

—job placement counselor could help C. find appropriate jobs, (because her verbal skills are good she is often placed in situations that require academic type skills and she fails). A job placement counselor could support C.'s finding an appropriate job, by helping her make applications, prepare for interviews and on and off the job follow-up until she and her employer feel she is secure.

—clinician working with a person with developmental disabilities should *never* assume that she does not have sexual concerns nor should the assumption be made that the client will initiate the topic. C. ought to discuss her sexual needs in her therapy sessions to insure her not feeling subordinate to her partner. Her feelings and needs expectations regarding her desires to have a marriage and children must also be explored.

H., subject #2, was verbally unresponsive to the first question although her aggressive behavior and inappropriate masturbation indicate concerns around this issue. H. did not respond to the questions regarding suicide but tried to introduce discussion about her brother's impending marriage. H. spoke of friends she has at an afternoon workshop in response to question # 4 but only briefly, then she returned again to family relationships and mentioned going to church with her mother. Inappropriately (or so it seemed) she then complimented the interviewer on her blouse. Then returning to her family, she spoke of a younger family sibling's boyfriend and that he spent a lot of time at their house. The interviewer asked her if her friends came to visit at her house and her reply was no. Her mannerisms throughout the interview border on very babyish to seeming to be appropriate for a 13 or 14 year old.

Issues: H. seems to be locked in an adolescent struggle with her mother and perhaps whole family. Afraid of disapproval and rejection she tried to meet her needs within the family but is unfulfilled and reacts with anger and by inappropriate masturbation (totally unacceptable in the Irish culture, in fact, Mother has talked of institutionalization due to behavior).

Clinician's Role: the therapy must be family and individual centered. It is not uncommon for the parent of the intellectually impaired child to hope the disability will be outgrown, this hope is difficult to give up and makes the child's adulthood more threatening to accept. Due to the conflict between the parent and adolescent it is not unusual for talk of institutionalization to surface at this time. The clinician must help the family see that H. is not totally dependent on them, she can have some independence with a community residence setting, she can work in a workshop setting, she is not only capable of, but deserves friendships with both sexes. Fears regarding pregnancy can be calmed by agreeing she is not capable of parenting and directing them to resources for appropriate contraception measures. If necessary, there is also opinion within the Catholic church that sanctions such measures for developmentally disabled persons (Bass, 1975):

—reassure H. that her feelings of sexuality are normal and give permission to masturbate in private.

—encourage development of age appropriate social skills via small group social interactions with inappropriate behavior a cause for removal from the group.

D., subject #3 was very hostile to any questions regarding her sexuality. She twisted her body further from the interviewer and finally replied to continued questioning, "you are driving me fucking crazy!" When questioned about feelings of despair she replied that she had been feeling angry and hopeless for about a month because she had changed cottages and now had to share a room. When asked directly if she had tried to kill herself she replied that she had cut herself up. D. did not know the meaning of the word therapy, when it was rephrased as sharing your sad, glad or mad feelings with someone who is not in your family or a friend she said that she used to talk to Father M_____, but she never sees him any more. When asked about friendships she replied that she had friends and she "would help out in the kitchen and cooperate." In fact she had problems getting along with the staff and other persons living in the cottage.

Issues: D. has a need to feel accepted (her declaration that she had friends when she did not)...she has a wall of anger around her to protect her from closeness, the very thing it seems she wants but cannot risk. D. cannot tolerate discussing sex, her strong reaction to this topic may be connected to her fear of closeness. Presently, she is difficult to like, D. needs to feel likable.

Clinician's Role: D. would be appropriate for a group situation on an ongoing basis with men and women. This would help her feel less threatened than she would in a one on one situation. The group should have a social orientation, i. e., activities such as going to the movies, card or board games, picnics, sharing records and meals together, etc. Interpersonal skills should be encouraged, support for individual needs i.e., anger, sadness, joy so that D. could begin to feel the value of being acceptable and part of a group. This would build D.'s feelings of self-worth and help her be a more pleasant person.

In conclusion, given the various living situations, intellectual abilities, and emotional stability of the three women interviewed leads this writer to speculate that what these women know and do not know regarding sex reflects the attitudes of the general population, i.e., regarding attitudes about birth control, masturbation, dating, marriage. It seems to confirm further that which most of us already know, sex is difficult for people to talk about. If this paper contains a message to the helping professional it is that the person with a developmental disability is a person first, with the same basic needs for love and acceptance that we each have. Their capacity for finding resources to help meet these needs is limited and women in this population are at particular risk. Given the appropriate educational and therapeutic environment a woman with developmental disabilities can live out her sexuality in a physically and emotionally healthy way within herself and with those around her.

REFERENCES

Abbot, J.M. and Ladd, G.M., . . . Any reason why this mentally retarded couple should not be joined together. . . *Mental Retardation*, April 1970, 45–48.

Bass, M. S., Surgical contraception: a key to normalization and prevention, *Mental Retardation*, December 1978, 399–404.

Bass, M. and Gelof, M., (Eds.), Sexual Rights and Responsibilities of the Mentally Retarded. Bass, 1387 Valley Road, Santa Barbara, CA 93108, 1975.

Miller, J. B., *Toward a New Psychology of Women*, Boston: Beacon Press, 1976.

Plotkin, R. and Gill, K. R., Invisible manacles: drugging mentally retarded people, *Stanford Law Review*, v. 31, 1978, 637–677.

Sletten, I. W., et al., Suicide in mental hospital patients, *Diseases of the Nervous System*, 1972, 328–334.

Sovner, R., Personal communication, March 1, 1982.

Sovner, R. and Hurley, A.D., Do the mentally retarded suffer affective illness? submitted to *Archives of General Psychiatry*, 1982.

Scheinkoff, S., Personal communication, March 29, 1982.

Smiley, C. W., Sterilization and therapeutic abortion counselling for the mentally retarded, *Journal of Nursing Studies*, Great Britain: Pergamon Press, 1973. v. 10, 137–141.

Weissman, M. M., and Klerman, G. L., Sex differences and the epidemiology of depression. *Archives of General Psychiatry*, 1977, 41, 390–405.

Wolfensberger, W. and Menolascino, F., A theoretical framework for the management of parents of the mentally retarded, in Menolascino (ed.) *Psychiatric Approaches to Mental Retardation.* New York: Basic Books, Inc., Publishers, 1970.

AN ACCOUNT OF THE PSYCHOTHERAPEUTIC PROCESS FROM THE PERSPECTIVE OF A CLIENT WITH A DISABILITY

Lisa Fay

There have been few disabled women receiving psychotherapy and fewer disabled women detailing their accounts. I offer this insight.

I went into therapy in 1979 not knowing what to expect. I had the assumption that those who went into therapy were "crazy," "nuts," or "flew over the cuckoo's nest." A professor at Framingham State College, my alma mater, suggested that I go into therapy after I told him that I felt violent and that my relationships were shaky. In short, I was unhappy with myself.

At first, I was reluctant to go in therapy because nobody in my family and only two relatives that I know had ever done so. It was something one never discussed or was encouraged in doing. However, I was relieved to know that many of my friends have been in therapy. One has been institutionalized and is now the mother of a daughter. It bothered me to hear my mother say that I went into therapy because my friends went, that I had subjected myself to peer pressure. The truth of the matter is, is that I went into therapy because I wanted to, even though I didn't know what it involved. My friends did not push me at all, and in many cases, they did not know.

I walked into a counseling center where I was assigned a psychiatric social worker who happened to be available at that time. I did not like the fact that I had no choice to whom I was revealing my most important thoughts. As a result, therapy was terminated after several months with no progress. Like we choose our friends and dates, I should be able to choose whom I see in therapy, not just any assigned caseworker. I had some bitter feelings, vowing that I would never attend therapy again. It took me three months to realize that I had a bad therapist, and that therapy can be beneficial with the right person.

In the meantime, I befriended a woman in the Information Center for Individuals with Disabilities (ICID) in Boston, a public agency dealing with

The author is a freelance writer in the Greater Boston area. She has learned to deal successfully with several disabilities including stuttering.

disability issues. She gave me the name of a clinical psychologist at the University Hospital in Boston. After much hesitation, I finally called him for an appointment, feeling that I had to talk with somebody.

I decided that he was suitable for my needs after a few sessions. He seemed empathetic to my issues, primarily interpersonal relationships and family conflicts. This psychologist also had training with disabled people, specifically their sexual needs. Every year he holds two conferences on Sexual Attitude Reassessment, emphasizing that nobody is too disabled to be sexual.

One may wonder why I decided to see a male therapist, and not a female one. I never thought the sex of the therapist made much difference, but I guess it does. I get along real well with my women friends; it is with the men that I have difficulty. I thought it would be better if I had a therapeutic relationship with a man so that I will feel more comfortable about having intimate relationships with men in the future. I will talk about this issue later.

In addition, not many therapists of either sex are trained to work with people with disabilities. It has only been since the 1970s that the disability movement has been in the public mind. Their early issues were education, employment, housing, transportation, and accessibility. Now the focus is more on sex education, and medical and mental health services.

We talked at length about my stuttering problem, a 20-year baggage. I told him that the worst part about being a stutterer is that I never know when I am going to stutter. This unpredictability is nerve-wracking and delays my personal adjustment and social growth in this fast-paced world. When I stutter, I am usually gasping for air like a panting dog. People react by walking away, ignoring me or avoiding eye contact. If people see a blind person or someone in a wheelchair, they stop to help them—with me, they are horrified. I hate terribly when I stutter on the most personal description of me, my name—and it is such a short one too. After I stutter, I feel like a ruptured sewage tank, leaking anger. What I really need is a hug.

My childhood was severely limited by defective speech. Other kids laughed at me, mimicked my stutter or refused to let me play with them—adults were no better. My mouth felt like an animal trap most of the time. The more I tried to open it, the more it slammed shut. There were times when I didn't talk for weeks, and my family always complained that they didn't know me. How could I tell them with such a trap for a mouth? Instead, I became just another mouth to feed at the table.

Ironically, anger gave me peace. I never stuttered when I swore. When I couldn't talk, I became violent. Throwing, banging, breaking objects, punching a window, and kicking an office partition are few of the many physical outbursts I and others attribute to not talking. My family always got on me for being violent.

My family has not always been receptive to the stuttering problem. They never failed to remind me that "if you can't say it, don't say it at all" or "thank God, you can walk." These messages still ring in my ears today. Their attitudes are no different than those reflected in society.

It is impossible for a family to understand everything anyone does. Even though my family may not understand everything I do or say, I have made it a top priority to have them understand the most important conviction of my life, and that is the value of communication. If they understand more, all the better. Friends take over what our families don't understand about ourselves.

It frustrated me the most that the people who were supposed to understand more about stuttering were sometimes the most insensitive. I tried to tell my vocational rehabilitation counselor just how stuttering affected my life. Keeping friends was difficult and my education suffered immeasurably, as I rarely spoke. I told him that without help, my potential as a writer would be forever limited as communication skills via speaking are absolutely essential. He turned a deaf ear to my pleas, saying that it wasn't a real problem since I never stuttered badly with him. That was partially correct since I had grown accustomed to him. But he never saw me in new social situations, schools, parties, and family gatherings, where I never failed to bomb.

I was beginning to wonder if I was in the wrong program. After all, Massachusetts Rehabilitation was obligated to provide services to those who have the most severe handicaps. If stuttering isn't considered a serious disadvantage, then I don't know what is. Nothing is so central to personality development as speech.

At first, my psychological therapist did not understand the emotional stresses of stuttering. He seemed to think I could stop stuttering, like turning off a TV set. He preferred to say, "You do it to yourself, Lisa." How can I be stuttering on purpose when I have spent 13 years in speech therapy or half of my life trying to stop it? Stuttering is like diabetes. There is no cure, only control.

I refuse to drop my therapist because he does not understand my basic conviction. He understands pretty much everything else. You just keep talking about it, and hopefully, we will reach a compromise. However, he is slowly realizing that the fun of companionship, the satisfaction of earning a living, and building self-respect come hard to those who cannot talk or have difficulty talking. Still, this dilemma does have a promising ending. I recently completed a speech therapy course at the New England Rehabilitation Hospital in Woburn where they emphasized the physical restructuring of the speaking apparatus. Treatment showed that if stutterers stayed within these new physical boundaries by producing a gentle onset of first sounds, taking a deep breath, and stretching syllables, then they decrease the possibilities of stuttering. I find this to be be true; however, it will take several months, possibly years, to be automatic. I now carry the attitude that I don't have to stutter anymore, and that talking is a better way of coping with life than violence. Talking is like having an orgasm; I never knew it to be this good.

Since I am talking more, I am finding out what a good person I am. I am not only a person with disabilities, but a person with assets. I am learning that I can be funny. So what if it is not as good as the JFK wit, but it is there. I use a larger vocabulary than before and words have more meaning for me. They are not tools for demands, but a permanent means of self-expression. I am now more generous with other people, I don't always have to know what they think about the way I speak.

Perhaps the biggest change in talking is that my relationships have become better. Men come to me more. Some were reluctant to see me because I stuttered a great deal before. I am feeling desirable and am enjoying dating to the fullest. I never knew life to be this good. It is like a curtain being lifted to remove any shadows. I am feeling better about staying in a relationship with men, and now know that a therapeutic relationship with a man isn't the only possibility that exists.

My other disabilities don't bother me as much as stuttering did. I can accept the fact that I limp a little when I get tired from a mild case of cerebral palsy on the right side of the body and that I don't hear too well. I only regret that I went through a large portion of my education with only one hearing aid when two were necessary to function. It has been since 1976 that I have been wearing two hearing aids, and with relief. My marks shot up after that. Before, the medical profession recommended putting an aid in the better ear. Now, if people have severe hearing losses in both ears, doctors will urge them to wear two aids to maximize the hearing potential.

Independence was also a big issue for me. Three factors delayed my independence from my family: chronic unemployment, various illnesses, and lack of readily available subsidized housing in Boston.

My efforts to obtain work with the Federal Government were futile, despite being eligible to work at a temporary position. I then signed up for a computer course which would provide me with a marketable skill in a tight Boston market. Even though I graduated from the program, I was the only one not hired. Even though I was never hired as a programmer, I published my first article in *Computerworld* about PROJECT COPE in April, 1979. I sent in the manuscript unsolicited and received a check.

Whatever other work I got did not pan out. In 1979, I decided that only one option was left, to go on welfare. I went on welfare to improve myself, undergoing a rigorous treatment of speech and physical therapy, and psychotherapy. I had many unresolved problems and realized that I could not become a productive citizen unless these issues were dealt with. I was feeling like the only option available was either jail or an institution, and recognized that I had better get myself into therapy before that ever became a reality.

The therapist helped me accept the fact that I needed welfare and therapy and he provided assistance in building a support system to help me through these troubled times. In addition to the medical treatment, I was able to continue my writing and get an apartment in Boston.

Even though I am still in therapy, I have learned much. Therapy has taught me that I have many assets. I am intelligent, attractive, sociable, and have fewer obligations than many women. I am single and have no children. I am also in the enviable position of working at the number one priority in my life: communications. In essence, I am not making a living, but am making a life. Although I have much to learn, I can honestly say that the favorite person I know is me.